PRAISE FOR *FOOD STORY*

"*Food Story* offers a roadmap to help quiet your inner a$$hole and reclaim your personal power. Elise guides you toward a new chapter in your relationship with yourself through food. This new paradigm is messy and beautiful, and it allows you to be fully human. It's the kind of book you'll pick up again and again, like your most trusted friend who never bullsh*ts you. This book is a treasure."

JENNIFER PASTILOFF
bestselling author of *On Being Human*

"Elise Museles has done something that few health experts have accomplished—she's created a powerful book about food and personal growth that's inspiring, practical, and full of soul. I consider this a must-have for anyone wanting to find healing and wholeness when it comes to their relationship with food."

MARC DAVID
founder of the Institute for the Psychology of Eating
and author of *Nourishing Wisdom* and *The Slow Down Diet*

"In *Food Story*, Elise Museles shows you how to heal your relationship with food, make nourishing choices, and feel 'in charge' of your health and your life."

MARK HYMAN, MD
New York Times bestselling author of *The Pegan Diet* and head of strategy
and innovation at the Cleveland Clinic Center for Functional Medicine

"I love this book because understanding your food story and feeling empowered to write it yourself is key to proper self-nourishment. Elise guides readers with warmth and compassion, as well as high-yield, actionable information and rituals."

DREW RAMSEY, MD
bestselling author, founder of the Brain Food Clinic,
and assistant clinical professor of psychiatry at Columbia University

"If you're looking for an authentic, practical, and delicious guide to rewriting your relationship to food, you've found it! *Food Story* delivers it all, and Elise makes it effortless and accessible. I want some of what she's having!"

ROBYNNE CHUTKAN, MD, FASGE
founder of the Digestive Center for Wellness and author
of *Gutbliss*, *The Microbiome Solution*, and *The Bloat Cure*

"Elise is compassionate, deeply insightful, and passionate as she helps us reframe our personal relationship with food in this beautiful, empowering guide."

KIMBERLY SNYDER
New York Times bestselling author, celebrity nutritionist, and founder of Solluna

"In *Food Story*, Elise shows you that grocery shopping can be fun, cooking can be simple, and eating can be deeply nourishing—both physically and emotionally."

FRANK LIPMAN, MD
functional medicine pioneer and author of
The New Rules of Aging Well and *Better Sleep, Better You*

"What's more delicious than the recipes in this book? The experience of finally having a loving, nourishing, and balanced relationship with food itself. Through her own story of vulnerability, honesty, and unmatched expertise, Elise Museles has written the ultimate guide to cherishing food and cherishing yourself."

JESSICA ZWEIG
bestselling author of *Be.* and
founder of SimplyBe. Agency

"I'm endlessly inspired by Elise's contagious passion and enthusiasm for eating psychology and how we can transform perfectionism and self-deprivation into simplicity, self-love, and peace, beginning with our plates."

VICTORIA ERICKSON
author of *Edge of Wonder* and *Rhythms and Roads*

"Ever wish you could turn the page on your eating habits and end up in a happier, healthier relationship with food (and I mean a long-term relationship, not a one-night stand)? Elise Museles shows you how to write your new food story and replace stress, cravings, and guilt with a sense of satisfaction and accomplishment."

"Finally, a book that helps you address your whole story and changes your entire relationship with food. Elise shows us how to rewire ourselves to eat and live with joy. I highly recommend this book to anyone who is ready to transform food anxiety and guilt and become a happier, healthier person."

"Something magical happens when we pick up a pen and write out our stories. Elise Museles has created a blueprint for releasing old narratives that keep us stuck and frustrated, resulting in fresh energy and a sense of personal power in this delicious offering. *Food Story* will move you into a beautiful, novel way of living, where stress is no longer a dominant character and ease and joy play starring roles."

"*Food Story* is an empowering book that takes us back to basics so that we can truly thrive. Elise offers essential multi-generational wisdom on how we can create healthy food habits for ourselves and, as parents, help build habits toward raising healthy adults."

FOOD
STORY

ALSO BY ELISE MUSELES

*Whole Food Energy: 200 All Natural Recipes
to Help You Prepare, Refuel, and Recover*

FOOD STORY

rewrite the way you eat, think & live

ELISE MUSELES

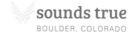
sounds true
BOULDER, COLORADO

Sounds True
Boulder, CO 80306

This book is not intended as a substitute for the medical recommendations of physicians, mental health professionals, or other health-care providers. Rather, it is intended to offer information to help the reader cooperate with physicians, mental health professionals, and health-care providers in a mutual quest for optimal well-being. We advise readers to carefully review and understand the ideas presented and to seek the advice of a qualified professional before attempting to use them. Some names and identifying details have been changed to protect the privacy of individuals.

Published 2021

Book design by Linsey Dodaro

Photographs ©Jennifer Chase

Printed in South Korea

BK06126

Library of Congress Cataloging-in-Publication Data

Names: Museles, Elise, author.
Title: Food story : rewrite the way you eat, think, and live / Elise
    Museles.
Description: Boulder, CO : Sounds True, 2021. | Includes bibliographical
    references and index.
Identifiers: LCCN 2020046358 (print) | LCCN 2020046359 (ebook) | ISBN
    9781683647195 (hardcover) | ISBN 9781683647201 (ebook)
Subjects: LCSH: Nutrition. | Health.
Classification: LCC RA784 .M874 2021 (print) | LCC RA784 (ebook) | DDC
    613.2--dc23
LC record available at https://lccn.loc.gov/2020046358
LC ebook record available at https://lccn.loc.gov/2020046359

10 9 8 7 6 5 4 3 2 1

To Steven, Noah, and Daniel
for helping me rewrite my food story

CONTENTS

Recipes & Rituals

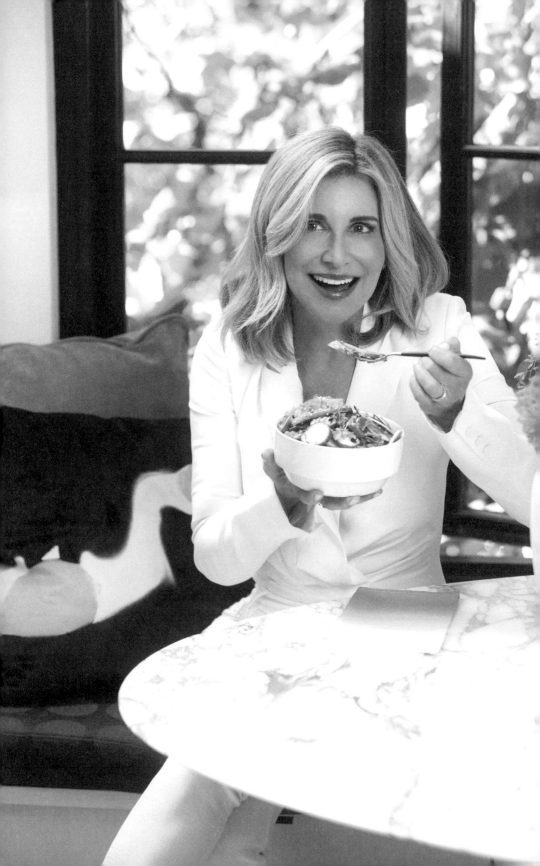

Once upon a time, when you were a baby or toddler, you ate when you felt hungry and stopped when you felt satisfied. There was no anxiety, no calorie counting, no self-criticism, no drama. Eating was simple and natural, and it happened without effort or complication, just like breathing.

Somewhere along the way, everything changed. No longer simple and natural, eating became confusing, exhausting, and frustrating. Suddenly, there were never-ending "food rules" about what you "should" and "shouldn't" eat, along with messages about body weight and how to achieve the "perfect" shape. Food became a source of anxiety and stress: What should I eat for breakfast? Why do I have so much trouble sticking to a plan? What is the *right* plan? Will this meal make me bloated? How come everyone else seems so at ease and I just can't get this food thing right?

If any of this sounds familiar to you, you're not alone, *and* you're in the right place. No matter how stressed, tired, and overwhelmed you feel right now and no matter how many diets and detoxes you've tried before, you can find peace and pleasure in food. You can eat in a way that feels good. You can feel comfortable and confident in your relationship to food. You can reconnect to your body and its inner wisdom so that you are healthy *and* happy. No guilt. No second-guessing.

It starts with understanding your food story, your personal narrative about food. How you feel about food and your body goes way deeper than calories or metabolism. Finding peace with food isn't just about eating more kale, drinking more water, or doing more yoga. It's about unlocking the power of your food story and rewriting the parts that no longer nourish you.

Because life is too short to waste time with food drama. You simply don't have hours (or weeks, or years) to agonize about food. You've got precious kids to snuggle, exciting careers to pursue, vacations to plan, dreams to follow, memories to make. When you have a distraught relationship with food, it steals your time, energy, and joy and takes you away from freely living your life.

I speak from experience. At one point, my food story was intensely negative—it was all about deprivation, rigidity, and control—and it almost cost me my marriage. The man who's now my husband got so tired of watching me obsess over every carb and stalk of steamed broccoli (no salt, no butter), he eventually declared, "I just can't do this anymore," and for a while, we broke up.

That's just one example of how a negative food story can damage your life. Food issues can harm your marriage, your career, and your friendships. Food issues can sabotage your mental and physical health. Food issues can make you a less-than-ideal role model for your kids—because your kids are always watching how you eat, how you talk about food, how you behave around food. They are soaking it all in, modeling themselves after you. (Even when it doesn't seem like they're paying attention, they are!)

Bottom line: when you've got a tense, negative, or just wonky relationship with food, it bleeds into every area of your life, often without you even realizing it. It's like a ten-thousand-pound weight that's bogging you down. That's the bad news. The good news is that when you view that relationship as a food story, you discover it's not set in stone. It can be changed. You can turn a new page. You can write a new story. You can start living differently and start feeling so much better.

WHY FOOD STORY?

I started my career as an attorney specializing in immigration law. As a lawyer, I learned about the power of storytelling. Tell a story one way, and you might lose the case. Present the story in a different way, with a fresh perspective, and you might inspire someone to change their mind, change a policy, or even change a law. A new story changes everything!

After practicing law for many years, I made a career pivot to follow my biggest passion: empowering people to lead healthier, happier lives. Even when I worked as a lawyer, friends and family often came to me seeking advice on all kinds of wellness topics, and eventually I realized, "This might be my calling." I became certified in holistic nutrition and eating psychology and launched a coaching practice to help people transform how they eat, how they think, and how they live.

When a new client came to me, I'd always start by asking, "Can you tell me about your relationship with food?" I hoped to spark a conversation, but instead I got a lot of blank stares, slumped shoulders, or clipped responses.

"It's too complicated!"

"I don't know."

"Oh, don't get me started!"

It was a dead end. Clearly, I had to rethink my approach. Recalling my training as a lawyer, I started reframing my question: "What's your *food story*?" Aha!

Thinking about their relationship with food as a story with major themes, plot twists, minor characters, and villains made my clients' conversations about their food-related thoughts and feelings much more dynamic, interesting, and energized. It gave them a new way to tell me about the foods they liked and didn't like; the self-talk running through their heads before every bite; their childhood experiences and memory-laden meals; the messages they heard about their bodies. With that prompt, my clients felt so much more open discussing their challenges and desires around food. With a food story, it was easier for them to see how their relationship with food wasn't only about them. Other people and outside factors play a role in it, too.

I began doing workshops about food story, asking friends and colleagues about their food stories, and you could see the light bulbs go off, with many people remarking, "I never thought about my food story." They started to understand why they had certain beliefs and behaviors, and they started to release some of the shame they felt. When they looked through the lens of a food story, they could see that, just like the ebb and flow of life, their food story was continuously evolving and changing. They weren't stuck on one page; rather, they were a part of an always-unfolding narrative.

I saw breakthroughs with my clients and healing on a whole new level. Once they realized that they could rewrite the narrative to support who they are now, they began to shift their mindsets around food. They were empowered to release patterns that no longer served them. They stopped worrying about every morsel on their plates. Food became a delicious source of nourishment instead of an ordeal. They treated themselves with more kindness. For most of my clients, discovering their food story eventually helped everything fall into place.

It can do the same for you.

WHAT'S IN YOUR MIND IS AS IMPORTANT AS WHAT'S ON YOUR PLATE

While spreading my message and supporting others, I was simultaneously unraveling more parts of my own food story. I had already come a long way and no longer felt preoccupied with the number on the scale. I was less fixated on "being skinny," and I had turned my focus to "being healthy." I knew how to feed my body the nutrients it needs to thrive. I was "eating clean," eschewing refined sugar, and filling my plate with the rainbow and the latest superfoods. I thought I was healed because I stopped obsessing about how I looked and paid more attention to how I felt.

But! Deep down I was still anxious. The focus of my anxiety went from finding the "perfect diet" to doing everything I could to "be healthy." Was I doing enough to be my best self? Maybe I needed more greens? More detoxing? More self-care? A better way to meal prep?! Plus I was putting a lot of pressure on myself to be an example for my young, growing family and to walk the talk for my clients and community. On the outside, I appeared to have this whole wellness thing down. Inside, I was worried about being the pinnacle of health and wellness and holding myself up to ridiculous and impossible-to-achieve (let alone sustain) standards.

I didn't recognize my thoughts and behaviors as problems, because they fell under the guise of "health" and "wellness." Ironic, isn't it? I was striving to be my best self, yet I wasn't feeling good while doing it.

As I looked closer at why I had made eating and self-love so complicated, I realized that I had the power to change my internal dialogue and edit the stories I was telling myself about what it means to create a healthy and happy food story. I worked to recall loving, supportive memories of food, like the joy of sitting down to family dinner every night when I was growing up and my mom's seemingly effortless entertaining that made holidays with my relatives so meaningful. I remembered watching my dad's unwavering commitment to taking care of his body as he headed to the gym each day and how he passed that dedication on to my brother, sister, and me.

I reminded myself of what food is really about: connection, nourishment, energy, pleasure, and *love*. I thought about all the positive things that food could do *for* me and stopped worrying about what it would do *to* me. I began to view my body as an ally and food as my most nourishing friend. I rewrote my food story so that my inside aligned with my outside: the conversation in my head was as supportive as the foods on my plate.

You likely picked up this book because there's something you're ready to change about your food story too. Maybe you want to quiet your inner critic and put an end to your same old monologue. Maybe you want to stop your pattern of starting over again every New Year's, every Monday, or every meal. Maybe you want to be able to enjoy a celebratory dinner (including dessert) and then just go on with your day without a stitch of guilt in your mind. Maybe you want to stop judging yourself for not eating (or looking) like the influencers you see all over the Internet. Maybe you want to let go of perfection and let yourself be human after all. Or maybe you want to do something completely different and finally allow food to help you live your best life, not interfere with and control it.

Whatever your reason, you *can* change your story. You can reconnect to your body and learn to trust yourself again. This is your chance to drop every rule, ditch every excuse, and look ahead into the clean slate that is your future. Your food story!

Okay, but how?!

PICK UP THE PEN

Now, it's your turn to pick up the proverbial pen and rewrite your food story. Think of this book as your personal coach offering simple, step-by-step instructions on how to navigate the often messy world of releasing ourselves from the guilt, shame, and stories we've held on to for far too long. *Food Story* is one part mentor, one part cheerleader, and one part friend who's there to stand with you every step of the way. It's a permission slip to love yourself, a way to get acquainted with the real you who's been there all along, and it contains the practical tools and recipes to help you get there, organized into two sections.

The Food Story Method

This book is about *you*. So if you're looking for a rigid plan, you won't find one here. Instead, you'll encounter questions for reflection, inspiring practices, and open spaces with lots of room to record your thoughts, feelings, and realizations. You'll also get all of the ingredients you need to banish negative self-talk, eliminate self-imposed stress, and reclaim your power and confidence.

You'll discover how to turn down the Food Noise and tune into the true expert of your body. (That's you!) You'll understand the exact steps to take to put your health at the top of your daily to-do list, rather than tending to one thousand other things (and other people) while neglecting your own needs. You'll explore how to be proactive with your food and mood, empowering you to take charge of your day. You'll get my secret to feeling and staying inspired even when life becomes messy, challenging, or overwhelmingly busy. You'll transform the energy and vibe of your kitchen (no new appliances necessary!) with a fun decluttering ritual that will change the way you feel every time you step inside it. Ultimately: you'll have all the tools you need to embrace and live your new food story!

Recipes and Rituals

Now it's time to cook and eat! After a lifetime of scolding ourselves for giving in to cravings or years of blacklisting certain foods (hello, carbs . . .), it might be hard to reimagine enjoying food again—enjoying grocery shopping, enjoying trying new dishes, enjoying eating—yes, deep enjoyment, excitement, inspiration, and fun! That's why I had to do something totally different so that you could experience food in a brand-new way. No, I am not going to tell you what to eat (although you will find a *lot* of plants!). Instead, I offer you a fun (science-backed) approach to look at food that puts you back in the driver's seat.

In this section, you will find dozens of all-new nutrient-dense recipes plus several simple rituals organized according to mood. Start by asking yourself one simple question: "How do I want to feel?" Happy, focused, radiant, strong, comforted, sensual, calm? Then you can choose a recipe, a ritual, or both to support the feeling you want.

Think: Bean Tostadas with Shredded Kale–Cabbage Slaw and Avocado for a boost of happiness. Glazed Salmon with Ginger, Lemon, and Tamari to keep you focused. An Eat Pretty Salad with crunchy jicama, slightly sweet pecans, and a tangy grapefruit vinaigrette to give you that radiant glow (side of Iced Raspberry Rose Latte optional!) Spice things up with a sexy Roasted Delicata Squash with Figs, Arugula, and Tahini Drizzle and Chili-Spiced Chocolate Tartlets to top off your meal on a sensual note. Or keep calm with soothing Roasted Root Vegetable and Chickpea Soup and a fresh batch of Blueberry Almond Muffins with Crunchy Nut Topping.

You can double the mood-boosting benefits with a dance ritual, a tea ritual, a writing ritual, a sunshine ritual, and even a cozy nook ritual. Keep asking yourself: "How do I want to feel?" Then cook, eat, and live accordingly!

BE THE HERO OF YOUR FOOD STORY

Food Story will guide you into a beautiful new chapter of your life—bringing you hope, optimism, and relief and restoring a sense of personal power. The past is in the past. The old story has already happened. It's time to stop stressing about food and step into a new chapter. Creating a new story starts with this book.

THE
FOOD

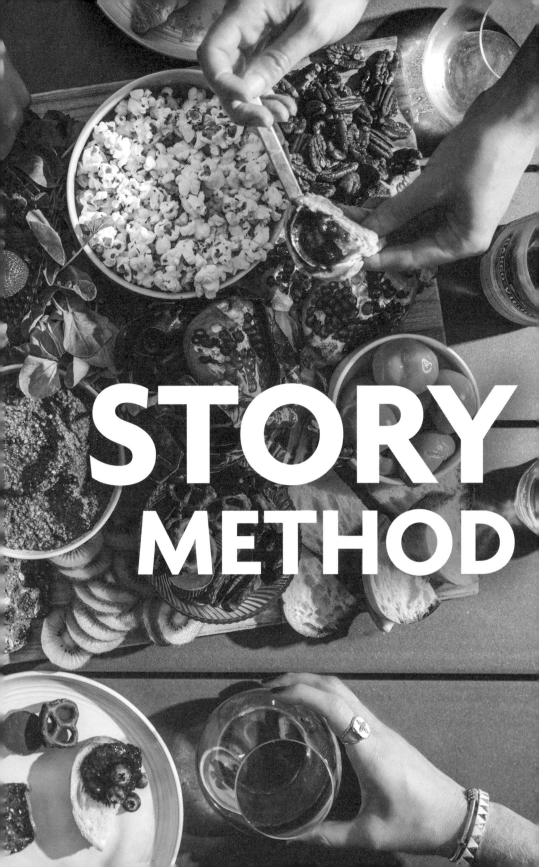

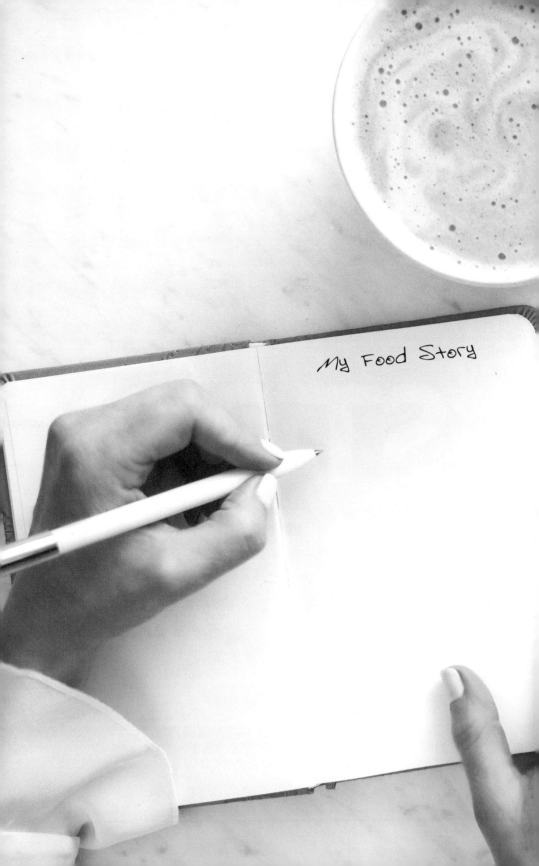

My Food Story

Part 1

DISCOVER YOUR FOOD STORY

CHAPTER 1

What Is a Food Story?

When it comes to food, everyone has a story.

The way you feel about food, the way you think about food, the way you deprive yourself or overindulge, the specific things you crave . . . there's always a story behind it.

Your food story might involve your mom, who congratulated you for getting straight A's by treating you to a hot fudge sundae.

Your food story might involve your dad, who quietly struggled with his weight for decades and who sometimes hid a stash of candy ("Our little secret, don't tell Mom, okay?") in the glove compartment of his car.

Your food story might involve your college roommate, the one who first introduced you to diet soda or laxative pills. Or maybe your favorite aunt, whose apartment always smelled like fragrant tomato sauce and whose hugs made you feel unconditionally loved.

Your food story is a big swirl of many things: the way you were raised, the messages about food you've received from your family and other influential people in your life, the advertisements you've absorbed from the media, your positive memories about food, your painful memories about food—all of it comes together to create a particular story.

Your food story = your beliefs about food and the words you say to yourself about food, either out loud or privately, inside your mind.

With food, you might be telling yourself a story about control and perfectionism ("I have to carefully track what I eat, otherwise everything will fall apart") or a story about confusion ("I'm just not good with food. I never know what to eat or how much") or a story about rewards ("I work hard all day long, so I deserve this margarita and nachos"). You might be telling yourself a story that makes you feel strong and empowered or a story that makes you feel miserable, anxious, and inadequate.

You might be thinking, "Oh, I don't have a 'story' around food. Not me." But that's not true. We *all* have a food story, including you!

Let me tell you mine.

MY FOOD STORY

When I was just a little ponytailed girl running through the heat and sunshine of Southern California, I had an easy, breezy relationship with food. I'd pluck oranges off the trees in our backyard when I felt hungry (or leave them shining on the branch when I wasn't). If I munched on a handful of bright jellybeans, my only thought was "Wow! Those were good jellybeans." I ate when I was hungry, stopped when I was full, and felt zero guilt about food. Then, early in my prepubescent years, things began to change.

It started when I was nine years old: I stood on a cold scale at the doctor's office while hushed conversation filled the space above me. I was there for my annual physical, but I was secretly hoping my mom and Dr. Gordon were discussing whether or not I could get my ears pierced, since I had been begging my parents for months. After I politely interrupted and asked if he could pierce my ears, Dr. Gordon turned to me and told me that if I worked very hard and lost just five pounds, I could come back to see him and get my ears pierced. I wanted nothing more in the world, and I nodded my head vigorously in agreement.

I don't remember much else about that appointment, but how I felt afterward is still fresh in my mind. I was eager to follow the doctor's order, please all the adults in my life, and earn my present. That very afternoon I started eating less, exercising more, and weighing myself religiously to the point of silent exhaustion. The numbers on the scale crept downward, and we finally scheduled the appointment.

When it came time to have my ears pierced, I cried: the pain shot through me like a knife. But I'd proven to myself that if I set my mind to something, I could achieve anything I wanted—including the number on the scale.

Around that same time, my father battled *his* own diet demons and good-naturedly padlocked the refrigerator in an attempt to curb his late-night snacking habit.

"Want anything before I lock up?" he'd call up the stairs to my siblings and me before wrapping a massive chain around the fridge, clicked in place with a ridiculously large padlock. The key went to my mom for safekeeping, while my sister and I discovered that there was just enough slack in the chain for us to squeeze our small hands through and remove string cheese or carrot sticks, our new favorite game.

The fun began to wear off when friends would visit and find the chained refrigerator, effectively blocking us from partaking in a pastime of historic importance: the late-night snack. I'd offer a sheepish explanation and usher them into another part of the house, silently fuming that my family couldn't be normal; later I'd arrange my social time to take place as much as possible at my friends' homes. Though the lock supposedly had nothing to do with us kids, it became a part of our food stories, which for each of us manifested in different ways: disordered eating patterns, shame, deprivation, embarrassment.

In my teens, I was constantly reminded to obsessively watch my weight at the all-girls' school I attended, where calorie counting and diet soda were as much a part of the culture as our matching uniforms and ambitious plans to eventually take over the world. During those years, I became more attuned to my mother's conversation with her friends, who maintained their enviable slender figures by pushing food around on their plates, bringing their own fat-free salad dressing to restaurants, and declaring certain food groups off-limits. I adopted their mantras as my own and then went on to dabble in more extreme forms of dieting. By the time I was a senior in high school, my friends and I followed a starvation diet to get ready for prom. Not even pickles allowed because "too much sodium," I vividly remember telling my best friend as I slapped one out of her hand—all that water retention and bloating! I also experimented with diet pills and what was certainly not normal eating.

These habits stuck with me throughout college and eventually made their way with me to the East Coast and law school, where I met Steven, the man who is now my husband. We hit it off almost immediately, eventually moved in together, and began to map out the rest of our lives postgraduation.

All of those dreams came to a grinding halt during what was supposed to be a special evening.

We're sitting at a fancy restaurant about an hour outside of Washington, DC. It's famous, world-renowned. The write-ups, the three-month-long wait for reservations, the artistic presentation of food . . . all of it creates excitement and anticipation that bubbles inside of me. I can't believe the day has arrived as we dine at our corner table with champagne glasses and two plates that look more like masterpieces than something to eat.

Except I'm not smiling. Or eating.

There's a lump in my throat and a pit in my stomach.

How ironic. All dressed up in the midst of a five-course meal with the love of my life, celebrating my graduation from law school, and I am unable to force myself to take even a single bite. He's discussing breaking up with me. Right then. Right there.

The reason? Food. Yes. Over food. We're in love, but he wants a woman who eats freely. A woman who can share his pleasure for chocolate and wine and wholesome, long, drawn-out meals, just like the one we are meant to be eating right now. More importantly, a woman who is present and fully engaged in the moment, not distracted or consumed by self-imposed rigid restrictions, like I am. Someone who isn't always on edge and anxious. We have all the other ingredients for a lasting relationship. We share a love for big dogs, hiking up steep mountains, dancing at loud concerts, reading spiritual books, and traveling to exotic places.

But there is the issue of the food. The damn food.

I've needed to control it for as long as I can remember, so fearful of what it will do to me. ("Will I gain weight? Feel bloated? Give in to my cravings?") Never in a million years do I even think that all of those anxious thoughts constantly buzzing through my head will cost me my relationship with the person I am possibly going to marry.

That night in the middle of dinner, Steven watches as I push cream sauce to the edge of my plate. He looks me in the eyes and says, "I enjoy eating and going to dinner, and it's important to me to be able to share one of life's essential pleasures. I don't get to do that with you. Never, ever, ever. You're just too worried about what you eat—or don't eat. You're rigid with all your food rules. I worry that you're going to make yourself sick. It's hard to watch."

The chef interrupts us. Not the waiter, but the chef in his white coat with his French name inscribed in the upper right corner. It's pretentious here, but that's the least of my worries. He asks, "Is everything okay? I noticed you aren't eating. Nobody comes here and doesn't eat."

Salt in an open wound. I want to scream, "Leave me alone! What I eat isn't any of your business." But nothing comes out except for the noise I make as I hold back my tears.

This scene isn't pretty, and this isn't some silly fight. This is deep.

Steven's words sting. Controlling food to maintain my weight had been my life for as long as I could remember. But I never thought it was a problem. I look good. I make healthy choices. I am fine with it. It isn't an issue *for me*.

I feel a chill when Steven finally stops me midsentence and tells me what he has been trying to say all evening: "Elise, I'm sorry, but I just can't do this anymore."

Food, he says, is a part of his life—and his *family's* life. He and I had discussed eventually starting one of our own, he reminds me, and he isn't willing to drag my dysfunctional relationship with food into it. He wants to enjoy our time together, not feel stressed out watching me obsess over carbohydrates, fat grams, and sodium counts. My stress is pouring onto him, making him feel anxious and on edge.

And so we break up.

After graduating, I moved back to California, where I threw myself into work as an immigration attorney—and began the process of healing my food story.

That dinner with Steven was a turning point in my life. I realized I wasn't healthy on the inside, and my complicated and messy food story was unknowingly bleeding into other areas of my life. This was a huge wake-up call for me. It was the first time I became aware that my consuming thoughts about food were not only disconnecting me from my body, they were disconnecting me from others, preventing me from being present and experiencing a life filled with joy.

I wanted eating to feel simple, not stressful and complicated. I wanted food to be a source of pleasure, nourishment, and connection. Just like it's meant to be.

Who knew a celebratory dinner gone bad could create such a revelation? But it did.

Looking back, I now see how my food story had been causing me unnecessary pain for years. The more I strove for control, determined to follow my strict narrative, the more it derailed my life. It was something I carried with me wherever I went, and it had a negative impact on everything—my career, my confidence, my relationships . . . and almost my marriage!

But here's the thing that I say to myself daily: "I'm never stuck. Whatever my food story is right now, it can be rewritten. I'm living proof!"

I have a new food story, one that I created, page by page. It's the way I comfortably embrace food and my body. It's how I connect with my family in the kitchen (my two sons love to cook). It's how I enjoy a date night with my husband at our favorite restaurant. It's inspiring thousands of women to peel back the layers and work on their food stories, too. Stress no longer plays a starring role. Now, my food story is filled with acceptance, gratitude, love, and FUN!

Most of us don't realize how deeply our food stories are impacting our lives until we take the time to identify and untangle them.

CHANGING YOUR FOOD STORY

When Vivian reached out to me to inquire about cooking classes for her family, she had her two daughters in mind. She wanted to make sure they had a healthy self-image and knew that this would be rooted in their relationship with food and their bodies. What she didn't realize was how her food issues made her a less-than-ideal role model for her kids—because her kids were watching how she ate, how she talked about food, and how she behaved around food and following her lead. "I hadn't even considered that my years of yo-yo dieting and current habits might affect my girls until you asked me about my food story," she told me.

Because when you have a negative food story, it can downgrade your entire life and filter into the lives of those you love most. Meals become a source of anxiety. You might feel preoccupied with intrusive thoughts about food. You can't seem to stop overeating. You feel out of control. You might feel ashamed about your eating habits. Or you might feel bored and profoundly uninspired about cooking for your family. Food becomes a source of pain and exhaustion, sapping your energy rather than nourishing you. The negativity seeps into your relationships, your career, and the way you parent your kids.

On the flip side, when you have a positive food story, it makes everything in your life so much easier. Grocery shopping feels inspiring. Cooking feels relaxing. Figuring out what to eat feels simple. Eating a meal feels nourishing and pleasurable. Frustrating habits (such as overeating to soothe yourself after a long workday) melt away. Food no longer has a controlling grip on your life. You are comfortable in your body. You just feel . . . good. When your relationship with food is joyful, your whole life feels different, not only to you but to those around you, too.

Now that you know you have a food story and are becoming aware of its presence in your own life, you can take the next step forward on the path to changing it: identifying your current story, the one that's looping inside your mind every day, possibly without you even realizing it's there.

Are you ready? Something tells me the answer is a big, resounding YES!

CHAPTER 2

Identify Your Food Story

When you look at your life, do you notice a frustrating pattern that keeps repeating? Is there a discouraging negative story you keep telling yourself over and over, day in and day out?

Maybe you keep repeating the same old story about *money*: "I'm terrible when it comes to financial matters. I always have been."

A story about *time*: "I'm always late for everything. It's just who I am!"

A story about *work*: "I can't afford to take a vacation. Everything at the office will fall apart if I'm not around."

A story about *relationships*: "There aren't any decent men in my town. All the good ones are taken!"

Or perhaps an old, discouraging story about *food*, which might sound something like: "I don't have any self-control when it comes to food." Or: "I've always struggled with food, and I probably always will." Or: "I know what I should eat, but I never do it." Or: "Healthy food is boring and doesn't taste good! I don't want to have to eat rabbit food like raw celery and kale for the rest of my life!"

We all have stories moving through our minds every single day. Some of these stories are empowering and help us to thrive. But others are not, and these can leave us feeling utterly stuck. Often, we repeat stories to ourselves without even realizing we're doing it. The story becomes deeply ingrained. Automatic. Like background music in your head, playing 24/7, guiding your daily decision-making.

Once you're aware of the fact that you're telling yourself a story, you can identify what your current story is—and change it if it's making you feel stressed about food, unhappy about your body, and frustrated, hopeless, and powerless to change your life.

The stories you tell yourself and the words you say to yourself directly influence your well-being and your quality of life. They have the power to change your mood—and change the course of your day. This isn't my personal hypothesis. It's backed by scientific evidence.

THE SCIENCE OF WORDS AND STORIES

Numerous studies confirm that words have a direct influence on almost every aspect of your physical and emotional health. Words impact your physiology (what's happening inside your body, including your metabolism and digestion), your cognitive function (your ability to focus and think clearly), your mood (how you feel about what's happening in your life and how you cope with stressful situations), and, of course, your performance (how well you're able to complete certain tasks, such as answering emails or planning dinners for the week).

The conversation between your own two ears can have a big impact on your success. Studies on the language-mindset connection confirm that athletes who talk to themselves in a positive, empowering way ("You've trained hard and you deserve to be here," "You're strong and powerful," "You're ready for this") perform significantly better in competitions than athletes who don't engage in such self-talk. Encouraging words lead to faster race times and more slam dunks, trophies, medals, and victories all around.[1]

Of course, it's all about the words you choose. Researchers found that simply saying the words "I'm excited" right before a performance helped people to sing better, hitting notes more accurately.[2] Singers who said, "I'm nervous" performed significantly worse—further proof that the words you say to yourself directly influence how your day goes!

The words we absorb matter too. MRI scans have shown that certain regions of your brain light up with delight when you hear your favorite uplifting song or when you read an inspiring quote or a poem that you love.[3] Positive words are like pharmaceutical drugs—without the side effects.

We know, without a doubt, that positive words and phrases have the power to improve your life. Tell yourself an empowering story, and with those magic words, you're setting yourself up for a healthy, happy, successful day.

Of course, the opposite is equally true.

Much in the same way that positive words can help you, negative words can harm you. Research confirms that verbal abuse during childhood can change the structure of your brain, creating a lasting imprint on the corpus callosum region.[4] That old saying "Sticks and stones may break your bones, but words will never harm you" is, unfortunately, not true. Words can, and do, hurt you. Negative words can literally leave a mark on your brain, like a verbal bruise. This damage can be undone, but it takes effort and patience.

This is why it's so important to be careful, intentional, and deliberate about the words you say to yourself. Every word you say out loud (and every word you say privately inside your mind) leaves a mark, for better or worse.

Your brain hears everything you say. Your body hears, too. It's always listening. No sentence goes unheard. If you say to yourself, "I'm terrible with food," your body hears that story of defeat and reacts accordingly. If you say, "I love taking good care of myself," your body hears that story of self-love.

What types of words do you say to yourself on a daily basis? When it comes to food, your health, your weight, your body, what's the predominant story that you repeat to yourself? Is it an empowering story? Or one that's disempowering? Is it a story that's helping you lead the life of your dreams? Or holding you back?

Many of my clients have never really stopped to consider, "What's my current story about food? What does it sound like? What are the specific phrases that I say to myself, over and over?" If you've never looked closely at this, now it's time.

EIGHT DISEMPOWERING FOOD STORIES

Through my work with thousands of clients and workshop participants, the women in my online community, and my family and friends,

I've found that many of us struggle with one or more of eight disempowering food stories. While these are not the only negative food stories (there are an infinite number of stories), these represent eight of the most common themes that arise for women of all ages, from teens to women in their seventies and above.

As you read through the following food stories, ask yourself, "Do any sound like me? Do these situations and phrases sound a lot like the words I think or say to myself?" You might discover that more than one story resonates with you.

Only by identifying the disempowering, unwanted food story that's been running through your mind can you change it into a new one that strengthens and sustains you.

1. The Story of Perfection
Similar Themes: Rigidity, Tension, Control,
Black-or-White Thinking, All or Nothing

My client Lauren used to put food into two categories: good or bad. When she ate what she perceived to be "good" food (kale, quinoa, raw unsalted almonds), she felt virtuous and proud of herself. When she deviated from her rigid meal plan and ate what she perceived to be "bad" food (potato chips, cupcakes, cookies), she felt miserable and sank into self-loathing. For Lauren, there was no gray zone. She was either being good or bad. She held herself to impossibly strict, unrealistic standards that no human being could ever possibly sustain.

If she wasn't being perfect with food, she felt like an abject failure. Her life became a cycle of restriction and deprivation followed by overindulgence, swinging from one extreme to another. Every Sunday night, she'd swear to herself, "Tomorrow, I'll start over. Starting Monday, I will stick to the plan. This week, I'll get it right!"

But when your plan is "Achieve unrealistic perfection," the plan never works out.

Inside your head, the Story of Perfection often sounds like:

"I have to stick to the plan, otherwise I will [feel like crap, gain weight, mess up my health, screw everything up]."

"I need to be more disciplined."

"I need more willpower."

"Ugh, I blew it. Today is ruined, but I guess I can start over on Monday."

2. The Story of Shame

Similar Themes: Guilt, Disgust, Hiding, Sneaking, Secrecy

When Nadia went through puberty, her dad didn't know how to cope. He made hurtful comments about his daughter's changing body, urging her to "cover up" her chest and insinuating that she was becoming too curvy and ought to lose weight. She was only fourteen years old. Her dad's behavior left a deep, painful mark on her spirit.

Nadia began to feel guilty about food and got into the habit of sneaking food from the kitchen back to her bedroom so that her dad wouldn't see her eat.

Years later, as a grown woman, Nadia still carried this story of guilt. Without even realizing why she was doing it, she'd often notice herself sneaking around with food—hiding candy in her desk at work, stashing snacks in her car's glove compartment, being furtive with certain types of food. Eating rarely felt like a nourishing, pleasurable experience. For Nadia it was always shrouded in a layer of shame.

Inside your head, the Story of Shame often sounds like:

"If people ever caught me eating this stuff, they'd think I'm disgusting."

"If people knew what I'm really like, they'd be horrified."

"I really need to get myself together. I'm so gross."

"I don't want anyone to know about this part of my life."

"I'm ashamed of myself."

"I feel anxious when I sit down to eat, and I'm not sure why."

"I prefer eating alone, in private, not out in public."

3. The Story of Confusion

Similar Themes: Information Overload, Overthinking,
Overanalyzing, Fretting, Worry

During our first coaching session, Roxanne burst into tears.

"I feel like I've read every book about nutrition that's ever been written. I've tried so many different ways of eating. I've tried to be vegan, vegetarian, raw, gluten free, paleo, keto, and a zillion other things. But nothing seems to work for me. I'm still heavier than I want to be. I still don't feel good. I don't understand why this is so hard for me to figure out."

For Roxanne, food had become a source of painful confusion. Even relatively simple tasks—like grocery shopping or preparing dinner for herself—felt complicated, overwhelming, and mentally exhausting.

Inside your head, the Story of Confusion often sounds like:

> *"I'm a smart person. I'm great at my job. I'm a great mom.*
> *I'm great at so many things. So why is food so hard for me?*
> *Why can't I just figure this out?!"*

> *"Should I be counting calories? Carbs? Fat grams? Or try*
> *intermittent fasting and for how many hours? There's so much*
> *advice out there. I don't know what's real and what's not."*

> *"I guess for some people, eating is easy and fun. But not me.*
> *For me, it's always a struggle."*

> *"I am so tired of the drama. I wish food could be simple for me."*

> *"I feel like 75 percent of my brain is constantly preoccupied with*
> *food. Thinking about it, worrying about it, wondering what's*
> *okay to eat and what's not. So much ruminating. It's so tiring."*

4. The Story of Escape

Similar Themes: Numbing, Soothing,
Self-Medicating, Reward, Avoidance

With three children, a demanding career, and a hands-off partner, Ellen's life was tightly scheduled and highly demanding. She'd be up at 6 a.m. getting the kids ready for school. Then she'd be slammed with work at the office all day long. After that, she'd wait for the kids to ride home on the school bus, and once they were settled at home, she'd dive right back into parenting mode without missing a beat—helping with homework, prepping dinner, cleaning the kitchen, folding laundry, reading bedtime stories. One responsibility, then another, then another. She rarely had a quiet moment to exhale and unwind. There was no blank space on her schedule. No escape from the nonstop carousel of activities. Except one.

Ellen's escape was a glass of wine, sometimes two (or even more), which she savored at 5 p.m. daily, like clockwork. "I need it," she told me emphatically. To Ellen, this was the only sweet, relaxing moment in her whole day.

Many of us often use food and/or alcohol to escape the pressures of life. You might use food or alcohol to numb out, to soothe your frazzled nerves, to transport yourself to another place and time, or to create feelings of comfort and nostalgia. This isn't necessarily a bad thing. Food and alcohol (in moderation) can, and should, be a source of pleasurable feelings. However, if you're escaping through food and alcohol too often—or if food and/or alcohol are your only forms of emotional escape—this can downgrade your quality of life.

Inside your head, the Story of Escape often sounds like:

"It's been such an exhausting day. I deserve this brownie."

"Work was a nightmare today. Do we have any ice cream at home? I could use a scoop. Or three. Or the whole container."

"My life sucks. People suck. Everything sucks. But margaritas are always here for me."

"Sometimes it feels like food is the only fun part of my day."

"When I get home after a long day, I make a beeline for the kitchen to get [a drink/a snack/a cookie]. It's almost like a compulsion. Sometimes, I feel out of control."

5. The Story of Not-Enoughness

Similar Themes: Compare and Despair, Self-Loathing,
Feeling Unworthy, Feeling Unlovable, Feeling Inadequate

Annika got a membership to a fitness club and visited twice, but then never went again. When I gently prodded to find out why, she told me she never has enough time to go. As we delved a little deeper, the truth came out.

"I hate going because I don't like being the most out-of-shape person in the whole gym. Everyone else there is super fit. It makes me depressed. So I don't go."

This is the trap of comparison. As President Theodore Roosevelt is famously credited with asserting, "Comparison is the thief of joy."

You might compare your career, income, house, car, marriage, skin, or physique to what other people appear to have—and then you feel worthless, like you'll never catch up, never measure up, never be as good as the sparkling, shining people you admire.

This can happen with all aspects of our lives, including food. Maybe there's an Instagram influencer that you follow. Her feed is a nonstop stream of images of positivity—she's leaping at the beach, doing yoga poses in the park, petting her adorable French bulldog puppy while holding hands with her impossibly gorgeous soul mate, and, of course, savoring perfectly styled superfood grain bowls and cold-pressed green juice in the sunshine. When you compare your real life to this impeccably styled Insta life, you feel like a hideous troll who lives under a rotting bridge in comparison. (Okay, maybe that's a slight exaggeration. Or maybe that's spot-on!)

Inside your head, the Story of Not-Enoughness often sounds like:

"I wish I could be more like [person's name]."

"No matter how hard I work, I'll never catch up to [person's name]."

"Some people have it all together. But not me.
That's just never been me."

"I've failed so many times when it comes to food. Other people can figure this stuff out, but I can't. Maybe I'm permanently broken."

6. The Story of Overwhelm

Similar Themes: Exhaustion, Burnout, Tiredness, Busyness, Constriction

Mia was in the midst of the most challenging year of her life. A divorce and painful settlement process. Selling the old home. Moving into a new one. Caring for a sick parent. One stressful event after another. She was courageously soldiering forward, handling each new crisis as best she could, trying to be brave, trying not to crumble apart. But she was completely exhausted.

"I feel like I'm drowning," she told me. "My to-do list never ends. I wake up, and I feel tired before I even get out of bed. Most days, I feel like I can barely breathe."

This sense of overwhelm crept into every area of her life—including food.

"There's just never enough time to go grocery shopping," she explained. "I end up ordering takeout late at night because I'm starving. It's not ideal, but . . . it just happens."

Never enough time to plan meals for the week. Never enough time to cook. Never enough time to take a Pilates class. Never enough time to meditate. Never enough time for a day off, an actual weekend, or, God forbid, a vacation.

When life feels completely overwhelming, many women begin to think, "Who has time for healthy cooking? For self-care? Who has time for a yoga class or a bubble bath?! It's just not realistic. Not with my crazy schedule."

Inside your head, the Story of Overwhelm often sounds like:

*"I never have enough time to take care of myself.
I wish I did, but I don't."*

"I'm swamped and can never accomplish everything I want to do."

"I'm so busy. I can barely breathe."

"I'm always slammed. My life is crazy. That's just how it is."

7. The Story of Later

Similar Themes: Postponing, Delaying,
Procrastinating, Feeling Undeserving

For Angela, life was put on hold until she reached her "ideal weight." She wanted to start dating again, travel more, and finally make that career move, but "now isn't the right time," she insisted. She even felt the same way about doing anything nice for herself, including updating her ill-fitting and outdated wardrobe.

"Once I lose these last fifteen pounds, then I'll treat myself to some new clothes," Angela told me.

"But why wait until someday later?" I asked. "Why not now?"

Why not invest in some clothes that fit you well at your current size? Why postpone comfort, pleasure, beauty, and happiness until some faraway day in the future?

When you tell yourself this type of story, essentially what you're saying to yourself is, "I don't deserve beautiful experiences. I don't deserve pleasure. I don't deserve happiness. I don't deserve to feel good about myself. I don't deserve kindness from others or from myself. Not now. Maybe later."

Would you ever speak this way to a child? Would you ever say to your daughter, "You can have a hug . . . later. Maybe"? Or "Change your body and then maybe you can have a dress that fits you"? Or "In a few months, maybe then you can play outside in the sunshine. Not now, though. Later"? You'd probably never say these things to a child or to a friend, yet many of us say these words to ourselves every day.

Inside your head, the Story of Later often sounds like:

> *"Later, once the kids are off to college and life is way less busy, then I can really focus on myself and my health."*

> *"Later, once the summer holidays are over, I will figure out a good eating and workout routine."*

> *"Later, once I fit into my skinny jeans, I will totally revamp my closet."*

> *"Later, once things settle down at work, I will start cooking healthy meals again. It's just been so crazy lately. But soon, I'll get back to it."*

"When I finally get this whole food and nutrition thing down, then I'll start dating again."

"Oh totally, I would love to take my family to Florida for spring break. But first I need to get bikini ready. Then I'll book the flight to reward myself."

8. The Story of Despair
Similar Themes: Hopelessness, Resignation, Defeat

Corinne was in her late fifties when she hired me. By that point in her life, she'd lost—and gained—the same twenty pounds about twenty different times. She had struggled with food her entire life. She had tried everything to try to heal her relationship with food. Books. Seminars. Therapy. Hypnosis. Sometimes, her approaches helped for a little while, but eventually she'd find herself backsliding into old habits.

"I can't believe that here I am, almost sixty, and I'm still struggling with this stuff. I thought I would have this figured out by now. This is not where I thought I'd be at this point in my life."

She wanted to feel ease around food instead of stress. She wanted to be able to just cook and eat and enjoy meals "like a normal person," as she put it. But after so many years of treading water, spinning in circles, and not making significant progress, she was losing hope that things would ever be better.

"I used to feel optimistic that I could turn things around, but lately, I don't know. Maybe this is just how I am."

According to the Oxford Languages website, the definition of despair is "the complete loss or absence of hope." Losing hope in your ability to change is one of the most dangerous stories of all.

Inside your head, the Story of Despair often sounds like:

"I try to change but it never works out. Maybe I'm a weak person."

"I'm a hopeless case."

"I wish I was stronger. But I'm not."

*"I'm so inconsistent. I make changes but
I can't stick with things. I'm screwed up."*

"I've tried so many times. I'm tired of trying and failing."

*"I just have so many issues with food. I always have.
I probably always will."*

*"I've been abused and mistreated in the past. I'm damaged.
I don't know if it's possible for me to change."*

Worksheet: Your Current Food Story

You just read through eight disempowering food stories. Which story or stories sound the most like your current situation? Circle the one(s) that resonated with you.

1. The Story of Perfection
2. The Story of Shame
3. The Story of Confusion
4. The Story of Escape
5. The Story of Not-Enoughness
6. The Story of Overwhelm
7. The Story of Later
8. The Story of Despair

Are there any other words or phrases you would use to describe your current food story? For instance, maybe you feel like you're stuck in a story about anger, guilt, betrayal, hiding, tiredness, busyness, distraction, boredom, inertia, or something else?

Let's continue exploring your current relationship with food. Without censoring yourself (this work is private, just for you), see if you can complete the following statements.

When I think about food and my body, I feel:

In moments when I'm feeling sad, stressed, or worn down, food becomes:

_____

_____

_____

_____

Whenever I can't resist my cravings for sweets, salts, carbs, or caffeine, I feel:

_____

_____

_____

_____

When it comes to food rules and nutrition, these are the thoughts that take up space in my brain:

_____

_____

_____

_____

A few less-than-healthy habits I know aren't serving me well are:

I feel guilty when:

I feel out of control when:

I become anxious when:

When I make a choice that I know doesn't serve me or won't make me feel good, I excuse my behavior by telling myself:

_____

_____

_____

_____

_____

If people bring up my food or eating habits, I usually respond with:

_____

_____

_____

_____

_____

Add anything else here that is surfacing for you right now:

_____

_____

_____

_____

_____

_____

Completing this worksheet may have been tough. But you got through it! I want you to acknowledge the progress you've already made to identify—and change—your food story. This is huge.

Now, give your mind a rest, take a few deep breaths, and know that you're moving in a beautiful new direction.

In the next chapter, you'll use the insights from this worksheet to help you dig a little deeper into your food story so that you can recognize the beliefs about food that are shaping it. Replacing old, outdated beliefs with new, empowering ones is the next step in rewriting your food story and feeling less stress, more ease, and more joy around food.

It might happen slowly at first, but then—like a snowball rolling downhill and picking up momentum—you'll notice that your new story becomes more and more vivid in your mind, your new habits become automatic, and food is no longer a source of agitation, worry, or discomfort in your life. You will get there. If I can do it and if my clients can do it, then you can do it, too.

Stories can always be rewritten. It's never too late to do this work. Just as you can always update your kitchen or computer operating system, you can always update the food story you carry in your mind.

CHAPTER 3

Recognize Your Beliefs about Food

E ver tried to refresh a flea-market furniture find by eagerly brushing on a new coat of paint? Right. Big mistake! Your pretty new showpiece is marred by a pockmarked, lumpy finish—that starts chipping off after a few days. Creating a lasting treasure means prepping and priming the surface first. Same goes for rewriting your food story. Identifying the story you've been repeating to yourself, perhaps one of perfection, shame, confusion, or overwhelm, is the first step. But for a new story to stick, you need to get at what's *beneath* the story, shaping it. Peel back the layers, and what do you discover? Limiting beliefs.

Limiting beliefs are negative thoughts about ourselves, our bodies, and our diet. They inform our actions and become the basis of our self-sabotaging behavior and our food story as a whole. They're fueling your patterns and eating challenges and keeping you frustrated, anxious, and stuck. Transform your limiting beliefs, and you reshape your thoughts and actions around food!

Even though your food story has been unfolding your whole life, chances are you haven't paused to really think about your specific beliefs. If you're just identifying them for the first time, you're not alone. Most people don't examine their personal beliefs about food.

But you need to understand what's limiting you before you can try to change it. So grab your detective hat and leave judgment at the door. Let's dig into your personal beliefs around food.

WE ALL HAVE LIMITING BELIEFS AROUND FOOD

Limiting beliefs can cling to us for a long time, sometimes since childhood. And whether you're conscious of them or not, these beliefs have created a blueprint that influences your daily decisions, for better or worse.

As a child, I was told to clean my plate because of "all the starving children in the world." It was a familiar line at our dinner table, one that I heard night after night. Even though my parents had good intentions, their words created an internal belief system that echoed for years to come. Whenever I didn't finish every single morsel and crumb on my plate, I felt guilty, wasteful, and extremely bad. To avoid those feelings, I'd eat my entire meal whether I was full or not.

I've shared this part of my food story in talks, on social media, and with my clients, and I've discovered that so many people grew up being a part of the Clean Your Plate Club. Even my husband still has a hard time leaving food on his plate because he heard that same message his whole life too!

There isn't anything wrong with eating the entire meal in front of you if you're hungry. The problem is that when you overeat because you believe you *always* have to clean your plate, you're disconnected from your true hunger signals. Not only does this limiting belief leave you feeling uncomfortably full after a meal, it may prompt you to mentally beat yourself up or start a negative spiral inside your own mind about your lack of control and willpower. Or you decide to punish yourself with exercise to burn off the food. You can end up feeling trapped in a destructive cycle. All from a belief that is no longer true for you!

While you may not have been told to finish all the food on your plate, you do have beliefs (many limiting) around food. We all do!

Those beliefs might seem like no big deal, but they run deep. You likely don't even realize how they are surfacing. But they can manifest in every part of your life, completely affecting your behavior and choices.

And they have staying power. Psychologists call this "belief perseverance." It's the tendency to ignore anything that runs against your beliefs and to cling to whatever makes them stronger. Even if they don't serve you!

Here are some common limiting beliefs about food:

"Calories in and calories burned are what matter most."

"If only I had more willpower, then I wouldn't crave things."

"Low-fat food = low-fat body."

"I have to deprive myself in order to be healthy or lose weight."

"I will be happy when I have the body I want."

"There is a perfect diet out there that I need to follow (and I need to do it perfectly)."

"Carbs are the enemy!"

"Healthy food is bland and boring."

"Losing weight is hard."

"I can't be trusted around food, especially decadent desserts, because I always overeat."

"I have a slow metabolism."

"Everyone in my family is overweight. Therefore, I am destined to be overweight, too."

"Eating fat makes you fat."

"Cooking takes too long. My life is just too busy."

"Food is complicated. I never feel sure about what I ought to eat, and I usually choose the wrong things."

BANISH THE BLAME

If you're struggling with limiting beliefs, I want you to know: it's not your fault. Having limiting beliefs doesn't mean anything is wrong with your brain. You're not weak or messed up for falling into familiar thought cycles. You're also not born with limiting beliefs.

The beliefs that have taken shape in your head were formed by a variety of outside influences, from your parents, mentors, teachers, and friends to your neighborhood, the Internet, the media, and diet culture. *All* of your life experiences up until now have helped to create your limiting beliefs. Blaming yourself for these external influences is dangerous for two reasons: it gives them even more power to write your food story for you, and it is—you guessed it—a negative thought in and of itself.

Here's the good news about all this: Your beliefs can be changed. No matter where your beliefs came from or how they formed, you can release them. Today. Right now!

CHANGE IT UP

You don't have to believe a tired-out tale. You can choose to believe something new. Why? *Because you're in command.* You are the author of your story and have the power to update your belief system at any time. It's never too late! Can you remember a time in your life when you believed something strongly—but then, much to your surprise, your beliefs changed?

For instance: Maybe you felt heartbroken after a breakup and started to believe it was your fault. You believed, "I'm not worthy of love." But then, after some time and reflection, your heart healed, and you realized, "Actually, I have so much to offer, and I'm worth receiving love, too!" With that new truth, you opened yourself up to an exciting future.

One of the most extraordinary things about being human is that your beliefs can and do change. You've experienced this type of change before. You can experience it again.

If you've been able to change your beliefs in one area of your life, then you can change your beliefs about food, too. The human mind is very malleable and capable of adapting at any age. The science of neuroplasticity confirms this, revealing how our brains are anything but fixed; they are capable of building new pathways between neurons (brain cells) every single day. We can rewire our brains and reinvent ourselves. New beliefs can take root and grow, just like a seed planted in a garden. This kind of change is possible for you!

Worksheet: Your Current Beliefs about Food

Now it's time to uncover *your* personal belief system. Once you've figured out what's limiting you, you'll realize how it's holding you back, and you can open yourself up to release what's no longer your truth.

As you begin to explore your current beliefs, use the worksheet in chapter 2 to remind you of how your current food story makes you feel. Pay attention to the adjectives you used to describe your current food story and relationship with food. Those descriptive words can help unlock the limiting beliefs driving your emotions.

1. What do you currently believe about food?
Write down some limiting beliefs that feel particularly strong for you—beliefs that you come up against pretty often. Look at the list on page 41 for some ideas to get you going.

_____

_____

_____

_____

_____

2. How would you describe your current relationship with food?
Do you feel stressed around food? Controlling? Inconsistent and erratic? Perhaps you feel confident and relaxed sometimes, then anxious at other times? Write down a few sentences that sum up the emotions you feel around food.

_____

_____

_____

_____

3. How would you like to feel around food?

Would you like to feel calm, liberated, stress free, confident, nourished, at ease, or . . . something else? Write down the emotions you'd like to feel. (We're going to dig into this topic more deeply later on—with strategies to help you get closer to how you want to feel!)

4. Have you ever experienced a significant change in your beliefs?

Write down some notes about a time in your life when your beliefs changed. Perhaps you felt differently about romantic relationships, friendships, family, parenting, money, work, or some other area in your life. What was your previous belief? What's the new belief that took its place?

5. Any other notes you'd like to write down?

Did this chapter spark any other thoughts or realizations for you? Write down anything else that you'd like to remember.

GETTING TO THE ROOT

Remember: *beliefs can change*. It's absolutely possible to believe something strongly and then later realize, "Hmm. Maybe that's not quite as true as I thought." Now that you've identified the beliefs shaping your current food story, you can let go of the ones that have been limiting you and establish new truths. We'll be working on that throughout the book. But I've found that so often shame around having these beliefs in the first place keeps us from letting them go.

We may know intellectually that our limiting beliefs have been shaped by all of those outside forces mentioned earlier and that it's not our fault we're carrying them around, but we find it hard not to blame ourselves. As a result, we stop ourselves from making the changes we truly want to see.

So what can we do? Go back to the time and place when our limiting belief took root. In the next chapter, you'll see why understanding how you came by your limiting beliefs clicks in place the last puzzle piece of your current food story, removes any shame or embarrassment you may have, and clears the way for you to turn the page and write a new story.

CHAPTER 4

Determine the Source of your Limiting Beliefs

f I could wave my magic wand and change one thing, I would end my destructive relationship with food."

That's what Nadia told me during our first meeting. (You met her briefly in chapter 2.) Her voice was weary and her demeanor, agitated. She couldn't quite sit still and seemed uncomfortable in her own skin. She looked like a woman who hadn't felt powerful and in control in a long time. Nadia also told me she was tired of feeling stressed by her behavior around food. Tired of turning to ice cream and french fries every time the slightest thing went wrong. Then tired of the self-loathing when she emotionally ate. And tired of having one half of her brain continually consumed with thoughts about *finally* getting this whole eating thing right.

Nadia would "eat clean," sticking to well-balanced meals comprising mostly whole foods. But the moment she felt stressed or upset, she'd binge to numb her feelings. Guilt would strike. She'd tell herself she was bad for losing control. Then another push: time to be good again. It was a cycle of extremes, one that repeated over and over, fueled by this limiting belief: "I can't be trusted around food when I'm anxious." She wanted nothing more than to change her behavior and stop the madness. And that meant replacing her limiting belief.

Limiting beliefs are at the bottom of our eating challenges and self-sabotaging behavior. In the worksheet in the previous chapter, you identified some of the limiting beliefs shaping your food story. Looking at that list, if you could wave your magic wand, which one would you most like to change? Which one is driving your most unwanted eating challenge right now?

Maybe the limiting belief "There is a perfect diet out there that I need to follow (and I need to do it perfectly)" is impacting your all-or-nothing approach to being healthy as you go back and forth between cleansing, detoxing, and the latest fads followed by periods of eating everything in sight.

Or maybe your limiting belief is "Food is complicated," and thinking about what to eat—or not—has quietly taken over your life. You obsess over every mouthful, every food trend. Meals are an ongoing source of stress, not enjoyment.

Perhaps you believe, "I have to deprive myself in order to be healthy or lose weight," so you count everything. Macros, points, calories consumed, and calories burned. Numbers control your choices.

You might think, "If only I had more willpower, then I wouldn't crave things" and be constantly consumed by guilt and beat yourself up for what you eat—or don't.

Or you just don't trust yourself around food: "I have no idea anymore what is best for me!" You've outsourced your inner guidance to some expert or influencer on the Internet who tells you what you should and shouldn't eat.

Do you see yourself in any of these limiting beliefs and scenarios? Or is there a different pattern that is true for you? (If you're stuck, return to the worksheet in chapter 3.) Once you pinpoint the limiting belief creating your biggest challenge, the next step is to ask yourself: When did it all begin?

WHERE DID IT COME FROM?

Can you identify the time when the limiting belief driving your unwanted habit, behavior, or challenge started? Is it tied to one particular event, tradition, or family belief?

Understanding where your limiting belief came from, or how it all started, can give you a feeling of relief ("Oh, *that's* why I always do that! It makes sense now!") and also release your self-blame for what happened in the past.

Your limiting belief might date back to your teens or young adulthood. Or even further back to age four, five, or six. You may be surprised by how far back your food issues go. We unconsciously absorb so much, including many of our limiting beliefs, during our earliest years of life. Before the age of six, our brains operate at levels below consciousness. We're massive sponges, taking in the ways our parents, caregivers, siblings, family, and community view the world. That includes their beliefs around food. At that time, we hadn't yet developed the critical thinking skills to question and consider those beliefs; our subconscious simply adopted them as our own. So don't be too hard on yourself! The good news is, now, as adults, we have developed the critical thinking power to revisit and revise them. No matter when your limiting beliefs took root, you can change them.

For Nadia, it started in her teens, when her body began to change. Her dad didn't know how to react, so he made passing comments to her about "being careful" and side-eyed her whenever she helped herself to seconds. He told her that because she ate too much, her body was becoming curvy. So eventually Nadia stopped eating in front of him. She would eat only in her room, sneaking in leftovers, bags of chips, soda, or anything else she could easily hide. Food became a crutch to avoid feelings of shame and rejection.

In Nadia's case, family was the primary source of her limiting belief, but there are so many people and experiences in our lives that impact us, often without us realizing how big that impact is. These are some of the most common influencers.

Family of Origin

Perhaps when you were growing up you received a message, however subtle, from your primary caregivers: your parents, grandparents, or other guardians.

As genetically similar as we are to our parents, we can also subconsciously inherit our caregivers' views and behaviors toward food and our bodies. Remember, until about age six we're incapable of doing much more than soaking everything in. Be honest with yourself for a moment. How many times have you caught yourself doing something and thought, "I never imagined that I would say this, but *I'm my mother . . .*"? So having similar patterns show up in the context of food and your body isn't too much of a stretch.

Back when you were a kid, how did your caregivers talk about food? Feel about food? Behave around food? What types of patterns or habits did you observe in your household?

You might have memories about special occasions, secret snacks, diets and weight-loss attempts, cooking together, or not cooking together. Some examples:

"I remember that Mom was constantly starting a new diet every Monday morning."

"Sometimes Dad would take me out for fast food. We'd secretly get hamburgers and milkshakes, and he told me not to tell Mom about it."

"My grandma loved to cook, and she was amazing in the kitchen! She loved to feed us. However, she would get really offended if you didn't ask for seconds."

Culture

We're not just shaped by our home environment. Our entire culture, other environments (school, camp, day care, sports teams, dorm, place of worship), and neighborhood affects us as well. The culture created by the people living closest to us influences how we think, feel, and behave around food. Society imprints upon us messages (both positive and negative) about how we "should" look, eat, dress, and behave that can stick with us well into adulthood.

Money

It may not seem obvious, but money and food are intimately connected. Your family's economic situation may have played a role in shaping your limiting beliefs around food. If your family struggled financially and food was scarce at times, you probably have a very different relationship to food than someone who grew up with overflowing cupboards. If money or its lack created stress in your household, odds are that stress informed your eating habits and view of food in some way—where you ate, when it was okay (or not okay) to eat, which foods were treats or rewards, and so on.

Friends, Mentors, and Other Influential Figures

It should be no surprise that the people we look up to could be the source of our limiting beliefs. These are people we want to emulate, and so we often, even unconsciously, take on their views and habits, including those around food. And no group, especially in our tweens and teens, influences us as much as our friends. Think about your closest friends from childhood, your teens, and your early twenties. Did you have any friends who were constantly dieting? Friends with eating disorders? Or, perhaps, friends with a really beautiful and positive relationship with food?

A Major Life Event

Your limiting food belief could be rooted in a big life event. Your parents' divorce. A tough breakup. A move to another city. Maybe it grew from some kind of trauma in your past. When we hear the word trauma we often think about clearly shocking or distressing events, such as sexual assault, parental neglect or abuse, the death of a loved one, or a car accident. But trauma can be caused by *any* experience that leaves us overwhelmed and vulnerable, and those can be subtle: a lock on the refrigerator, a stupid boy offhandedly saying how much he loves skinny girls, a ballet teacher criticizing your body, an aunt denying you a piece of cake. These may not sound like major life episodes, but any of these moments could be the traumatic event in your story that prompted you to turn to food for comfort or restrict food to help you feel in control. No incident is unimportant when you are searching for the origins of your limiting beliefs.

LOOK WITH LOVE

In this chapter's worksheet, you'll work through your memories about food to find the role it has played in your life and the origins of your limiting beliefs.

It's important to understand how you came to have your limiting beliefs and the ways these pivotal influences have shaped your food story. But look through your past with love, not judgment. Forgive yourself. Forgive your parents and other important people in your life. Nadia wrote her father a letter so she could release some of her resentment and lingering shame, and even though she never gave it to him, the process of setting those powerful words down on the page was crucial. It allowed her to move forward. It allowed her to change. Forgiveness can help you do the same.

Worksheet: The Sources of Your Limiting Beliefs

It's one thing to think about the past, but doing so with a pen in hand is an entirely different experience. In this exercise, you'll dive deep, identifying experiences and relationships that shaped your limiting beliefs and your current food story.

1. Family of origin
What do you remember about food and your family? Write down a few memories that come to mind.

_____

_____

_____

_____

_____

Overall, what kinds of messages about food did you receive from your family? Any positive messages that you'd like to retain and keep in your life? Any negative messages that you'd like to release?

_____

_____

_____

_____

_____

_____

2. Culture

Growing up, what was your culture, environment, or neighborhood like? What kinds of people lived nearby, and how did they think, feel, and behave around food?

Overall, what kinds of messages about food did you receive from your culture? Any positive messages that you'd like to retain and keep in your life? Any negative messages that you'd like to release?

---

3. Money

Write down a few memories about food and money that come to mind.

Overall, what kinds of messages about food and money did you receive during your childhood and early adulthood? Any positive messages that you'd like to retain and keep as part of your story? Any negative messages that you'd like to release?

4. Friends, mentors, and other influential figures

Overall, what kinds of messages about food did you receive from your friends in childhood and early adulthood? How about mentors or other influential figures? Any positive messages that you'd like to retain and keep as sacred to your story? Any negative messages that you'd like to release?

Think about the people closest to you today, including colleagues, mentors, friends, or anyone else who influences your life. What kinds of messages about food do you receive from your current circle? Positive? Negative? Both?

_____

_____

_____

_____

_____

_____

_____

5. A major life event

Do you think a major life event is connected to your limiting beliefs and food story? If so, in what ways?

_____

_____

_____

_____

_____

_____

_____

KEEP WHAT NOURISHES, RELEASE WHAT DOESN'T

Changing your food story doesn't mean that you have to completely erase your past and start from scratch. You don't have to remove those parts from your memory. You can use your discernment and choose to hold on to some parts while releasing others.

Perhaps you remember enjoying special holiday meals with family gathered around the table as a kid. You have fond memories of these celebrations, and you'd like to continue this tradition with your own family. That's great!

Maybe you also remember watching your dad struggle intensely with alcohol and overeating—and that's *not* a pattern that you want to carry forward in your own life. That's a great observation, too.

Just like an editor working on a book, you get to decide which parts of your current food story you want to keep and which parts to remove or revise.

Keep the parts that nourish you, the parts you love and cherish.

Anything that doesn't feel nourishing, you can choose to let go.

The journey of rewriting your food story is one of healing, and healing starts with awareness. Over the last several chapters, you've become more aware of the themes driving your current food story, the limiting beliefs shaping it, and the origins of those limiting beliefs. You have all you need to turn the page and begin the process of releasing what no longer serves you.

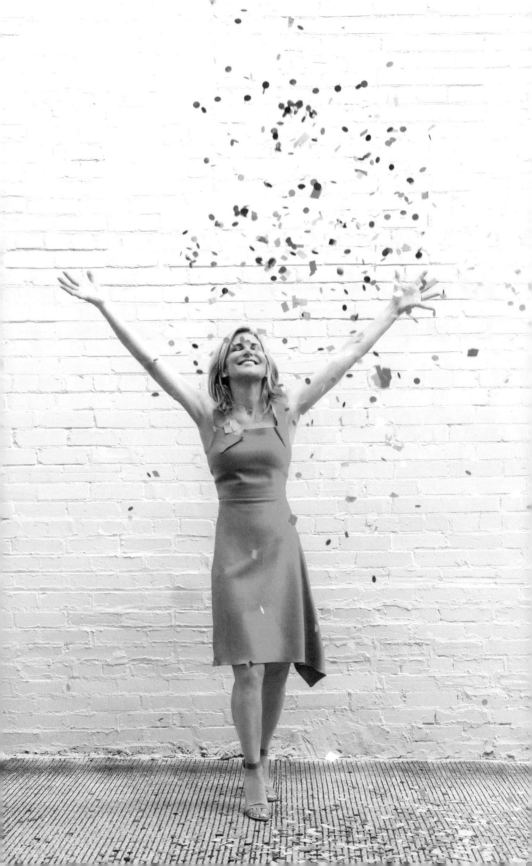

Part 2

RELEASE WHAT NO LONGER SERVES YOU

CHAPTER 5

Release Your Old Food Story

nly by shaking off the old, outdated patterns weighing us down can we step forward and create the kind of change that is meaningful and freeing. One of the most powerful ways to do this? Write them down. Writing is an incredible release. Those of you who regularly journal know what I mean! Even if that's not you, I'm sure you've felt the sweet relief that comes from simply jotting down your to-do list and pinning your tasks in black and white instead of allowing them to occupy space in your mind. Converting thoughts to words on a page makes them more real somehow and more manageable. Writing not only helps us organize our thoughts, it can help us understand our experiences and feelings in a completely new and unexpected way. Writing your current food story is like pouring out stagnant water to make space for a new flow—and a new story. And sharing our stories reminds us that we're not alone on this journey.

In 2012, I was getting my certification in eating psychology, and as part of the program, I had to complete writing assignments about my personal relationship with food. Over the several years I'd spent healing old stories and changing my narrative, I had never actually written down a single word about my struggles and challenges. And, wow, writing it all down proved to be powerful. My truths rapidly emerged with potent new clarity before my very eyes. In this physical process of moving my hand across the page, I realized something huge that had been keeping me consumed and held back for too long: my food story was a story my own brain had made up.

You see, there were years I'd gripped onto the false belief that somewhere existed a perfect diet. And that this so-called perfect diet would lead to a flawless body. And that having that flawless body would inevitably lead to long-term happiness. It was only through writing my story down that I was able to understand how terribly paralyzing this embedded belief had been for me all that time, keeping me stuck and honestly quite miserable, like I was always holding my breath. I wasn't thriving by carrying this thought, and I would never be able to be my most vibrant self until I released it. When I did, it was a massive exhale.

Somehow, shortly after, I mustered enough courage to share my discoveries in a blog post for a popular website. Of course, nowadays everyone is discussing the benefits of vulnerability, but back then people weren't as open about their personal struggles online. Sharing your raw truth wasn't part of the collective conversation.

I reread my post about two hundred times (hello again, perfectionist!) and remember actually feeling my hands tremble as I hit publish. Much to my surprise, the response was amazingly positive! Readers from everywhere immediately reached out to say how much my story resonated and then opened up about their own difficulties. It was a wake-up call that maybe *nobody*'s perfect and that I definitely needed to let go of my ongoing and unattainable quest for total control, because it was only a road to nowhere. Since then, I use writing and sharing as essential tools in the development of my own evolving food story, and I encourage you to do the same.

WRITE IT DOWN

So why bother writing your food story down? Well, writing helps you to see experiences and events in a new way. You may be surprised at how different your written reflections are from the ones swirling in your memory. Writing enables you to organize your thoughts and insights and make meaning from them more easily than if you just mull them over in your head. I might not ever have been able to identify the underlying limiting belief at the core of my food story if I hadn't taken the time to hash it out on the page. Writing allows you to slow down, pay attention, and make sense of the past.

Words are powerful, and they move energy through us, like breathing. Yes, writing is energizing! And best of all, when you put something in writing you're far more likely to take action. When you actually see your story on paper (or your screen), it becomes physically real and moves you toward holding yourself accountable for changing it.

As you write, you'll probably dig up some truths that might initially make you a little uncomfortable. That's perfectly okay. Allow yourself to feel your feelings without judgment or attachment. Looked at in this way, they can teach you profound things about yourself while shedding light on all those old ideas that have been clouding and disrupting your vision. Keep your eyes fixed on the bigger picture: you're getting closer to writing your new food story.

SHARE YOUR FOOD STORY

Writing down your food story is a cathartic step. Of course, you can always keep it private. However, if you do feel brave enough to share your story with someone else, it can take you a step further toward a powerful transformation. Why? Because when you share something that you've felt ashamed about—something you've hidden for a long time, like your struggles with food—it feels like a thousand pounds being lifted off your chest. Shame is such a heavy, exhausting emotion. It limits us, keeping us stuck in a tight, cramped way. It presses down on us so we can't sleep, live, or grow. Shame can be so paralyzing because you may not even realize an invisible weight is affecting you—until you write your story, share it, and set it free.

While it might feel a little scary (or, let's be honest, completely terrifying!) to expose an untold piece of your story out loud, it's a huge opportunity for release. And, most importantly, it will help you feel connected—connected to yourself, the person you share it with, and, of course, your inner wisdom.

The first time I felt brave enough to publicly share my food story in person, I was the keynote speaker at a wellness event, standing in a room full of 150 people. I took a deep breath, then spoke candidly about my relationship with food and how reflecting on an entire lifetime's worth of meals had helped to inform and redirect my path. I pulled my pain and words out from deep inside me, and by the end I felt raw.

And then . . . there was silence.

Like, pin-drop, record-skip, deafening silence.

"Do they all think I'm crazy?" I wondered. All my years of self-doubt, perfectionism, and food guilt came rushing back, flooding the space inside of me I had just emptied.

Then a woman named Lila raised her hand. She admitted that she didn't like sitting down at the dinner table with her husband and children and she couldn't understand why. Her guilt around her inability to enjoy a meal with her family had nagged at her for years, especially when she thought of her three young kids. But when she heard my story, even though it had nothing to do with hers, she was immediately inspired to reflect on her own.

Suddenly, Lila connected the dots and realized that her childhood dinner table had been more fraught than friendly because of an alcoholic father and a diet-obsessed mother. She found the thread, stitched way back in her past, that still influenced her food story years later. By understanding it, she became empowered to lift the veil of shame and change her entire narrative.

That day, the magic happened—a room full of women felt inspired to stand up and share snippets of their own food stories. We realized that we weren't alone in our struggles. Our food stories, however disparate, connected us to the deepest parts of ourselves *and* to each other.

You don't have to stand onstage in front of an audience. Sharing your story with even one person can be poignant and healing. I gave a talk about food stories in a yoga studio, and soon after I received an email from a man whose wife had been in the audience. He wrote, "Naomi just came home and told me her food story for the first time!" After ten years of marriage, they'd entered a new chapter where they could talk about their struggles with food and support each other. Sharing not only helps you heal, it strengthens relationships with the people you love most.

Hearing your story can be the permission slip others need to raise their hands and say, "Hey, I've struggled with this stuff too . . ." Wherever I share about my food story, people end up feeling moved to share theirs—on social media and my blog, on podcasts, and in front of live audiences. Right there, on the spot!

You can talk to those you love about what they're struggling with and let them know you are there for them, too. Simply by asking your partner, your best friend, your sister, or anyone you care about, "What are your food issues?" you're sending a signal that food stories don't have to be secretive and shameful.

These conversations might not come easily, and that's natural. Many of us have spent years, even decades, feeling embarrassed about our food and body struggles. But I can tell you from experience that when I created an environment where I could talk openly about my complicated and messy relationship with food, I felt supported, seen, and inspired to change.

Whom should *you* talk to? It may be your partner, a trusted friend, a therapist, or someone else whom you feel emotionally safe being around. Counterintuitively, sometimes we open up to total strangers, because anonymity helps us to feel a bit less scared. Remember the last time you shared something unexpectedly personal with your seat mate on an airplane? I'm sure at some point we have all done it! Whomever you choose, take a deep breath and allow your words to tumble out. We all deserve to feel seen and heard, and opening up about your story is a means to release emotions that block you from experiencing joy.

Sharing Dos and Don'ts

- Do be cautious with social media. You're putting yourself out there in a big way, so make sure you're comfortable going public with information that is very personal.

- Don't be surprised if someone goes negative on you. There's always one (or more!) who does. Focus on the support and leave the rest.

- Do choose a suitable time and place.

- Don't assume now is the right time for a heart-to-heart. Check in with your desired listener and find some uninterrupted space in your day when both of you can be calm and attentive.

- Do be honest if you're feeling nervous. That's natural!

- Don't be afraid of scaring them off. You are stepping into your power and lightening your load just by sharing your story, no matter what the reaction.

- Do give your listener time to respond.

- Don't expect them to share their feelings or feedback right away—or at all! They may want some time to digest all that you've said and reconnect with you about it in their own way and time, or not. That's okay. The point is, you've been heard.

YOUR STORY MATTERS

Writing and talking about your food story enables you to free yourself from the past. It's a very powerful thing to know that you're not alone in your anxiety or pain. The more we share our stories, the more we normalize these conversations. And if you're thinking that your food story isn't that interesting or is too messy or extremely embarrassing or [fill in the blank], please stop yourself right now. If there is one thing that I want you to take away from this chapter, it's that *your story matters* . . . thinking about it, writing about it, and talking about it. This is how you heal, and this is how *we* heal together.

Worksheet: Write and Share Your Current Food Story

A quick reminder that your current food story is exactly that—a story! Stories are not set in stone. They are fluid.

PUTTING YOUR STORY ON THE PAGE

Later in this book, you'll have the opportunity to write down all the details about your *new* food story—the positive, empowering story that you're excited to dive into! But for this exercise, please focus on your present-day story.

As you're working through the prompts, here's a statement that might help you get into the right mindset: "This is my current food story, but it doesn't have to be my story going forward. I can adopt new beliefs. I can learn new skills. When it comes to making choices about food and my health, I can learn to be proactive rather than reactive. I own my past and appreciate the lessons learned—and I recognize that I can change now."

If you're thinking, "But I'm not a good writer!" no worries. The following worksheet is designed to make it easy, and you've already done a crucial part of the work. In the past few chapters, you dug deep, identifying your food story themes and limiting beliefs and exploring the memories, circumstances, and experiences that contribute to your relationship with food. Refer back to the work you've done on previous worksheets to refresh your memory.

Or don't! There's absolutely no wrong way to write out your story. I recommend writing your story out by hand, as some research suggests doing so helps us process and understand the material better than when we write electronically, but just follow your instincts![1] Great writing is really about telling the truth from your body. Don't feel as if you have to fill in every single blank; what to include—or not—is totally up to you.

MY CURRENT FOOD STORY

by: _____

I was born in _____ and raised by _____ .
As a child, my parents/caregivers had a _____ relationship
with food. I grew up watching them do things like _____
_____ , which often caused me to
feel _____ .

From my childhood, teen years, and early adult life, one negative
memory I have about food is _____
_____ . One positive
memory I have about food is _____ .

Many factors—including my family of origin, friends, mentors, my
cultural and economic reality, the media, and generational trauma—
have all shaped my current beliefs about food.

Currently, when it comes to food, I believe/I often notice myself
thinking things like _____
_____ .

I recognize that some of these beliefs may not be helpful or even true.

Currently, when it comes to food, I often engage in behaviors that
I'd like to release, such as _____
_____ .

I recognize that I have the power to change these patterns.

Overall, when it comes to food, I feel _____

_____. I'm tired of _____

_____. I don't enjoy _____

_____.

I take responsibility for my current food story. I understand that the only person who can change my story is *me*.

I get to decide which parts of my story I want to keep and carry forward into the future and which parts I want to change or release.

I forgive my parents/caregivers for _____

_____.

I know they never meant to harm me. They were doing their best with the knowledge and resources they had.

I forgive myself for _____

_____. I, too, was just doing my best.

I understand that forgiveness is a gift from myself to myself. It's a gift that helps me feel emotionally lighter. With forgiveness, I'm unburdening myself so that beautiful changes can happen more quickly.

Going forward, I'm excited to give my body the love and attention that it deserves. I'm excited to step into a new relationship with food, cooking, and my health and well-being.

I'm excited to try _____

_____.

I'm excited to start believing/thinking _____

_____.

And I'm excited to feel _____

_____.

One of the bravest and most empowering ways to begin rewriting your story is to share it, in whatever setting you feel most comfortable: one-on-one, in a group, on social media.

How would you feel most comfortable sharing your story?

_____

_____

_____

_____

_____

_____

What steps do you need to take to make it happen?

_____

_____

_____

_____

_____

_____

CHAPTER 6

Quiet the Food Noise

will never forget my first marathon, but not in the way you might think . . .

I trained for months and months, doing all the things you do leading up to an endurance event. With one exception: I wasn't eating the food my body needed. I knew other runners who loaded up on carbs before their runs, and while secretly I thought that sounded divine, I wouldn't allow myself to follow suit.

As someone who stayed up on the latest and greatest in the wellness industry before even becoming a health coach, I was up to speed on food conversations, and I knew the trend at that time: low carb! Magazines were writing about it. My friends were talking about it. Everyone was vilifying carbs.

So even though my body was nudging me to join those all-you-can-eat pasta parties my running buddies were hosting, I ignored the nudge and thought I knew better than everyone else, vehemently sticking to my low-carb plan.

The big day came. I was so excited. I had my own cheering section—my boys and husband waving and shouting from the sidelines. My dad even surprised me and flew to DC from California to see me run.

The starting gun went up, and then—BANG! I was off, feet pounding, heart thumping. I was going strong and making good time. But it wasn't long before I realized something was wrong.

My body felt heavy. My muscles were overextended. The run got tougher, and it became harder for me to push through. Then, at mile seventeen, I just stopped. I literally couldn't move. I wasn't seeing straight. I'd hit the wall. And my body didn't have the fuel it needed to keep going.

I vaguely remember grabbing a cookie from an outstretched hand and somehow making it across the finish line. Barely. Right away I knew this was all because of my nutrition—or lack thereof! I hadn't been eating for performance, like a runner should. I hadn't been listening to my body along the way to the big day. I was too distracted by what I now call Food Noise.

WHAT IS FOOD NOISE?

Food Noise is a dangerous kind of villain, because it's everywhere and it's often difficult to recognize. And its nefarious endgame? To distract you from listening to your body and what it needs to feel nourished.

You know those magazine ads for the latest "superfood" you have to start eating if you want to be healthy? Or the documentary about how sugar is killing you? Or the headlines about bikini bodies, New Year New You, or anything that makes you feel that you aren't good enough exactly as you are? That's Food Noise.

Or what about that running commentary in your head? The one that starts up every time you pick up your fork or think about your next meal, telling you to listen to what you heard about, "Eat this, not that." Instructing you to follow all of those food rules and then reminding you to feel guilty whenever you break those rules. That's Food Noise, too.

Food Noise is what you hear *in the moment* that affects your choices, your habits, and your self-esteem. We've talked a lot about limiting beliefs, those seemingly ingrained convictions about food that have shaped your current food story. Their source is often rooted in the past, and you've done some hard work looking back to determine where those limiting beliefs came from so you can change them. With Food Noise, we're right here, right now, in the present. On the surface,

Food Noise can seem harmless—what's so terrible about new super-foods or the benefits of time-restricted eating? Well, nothing, on their own. But daily Food Noise can become a loud chorus that confuses and disempowers you.

My client Amanda came to my office because she knew something was wrong, and the problem kept getting worse. She was beyond exasperated. "I'm just trying to get this food thing right," she told me. A smart, successful lawyer, Amanda had a mind for details. She wanted to nourish her body with healthy food and to make informed decisions about what she ate. So she did what she knew best and researched everything. She gathered as much information as she could. For every food, she'd find all sorts of articles, studies, and expert opinions.

The problem was, things rarely lined up.

A respected food blogger would post, "Eat fish, it's so good for you!" But a quick Google search later, Amanda would pull up an article about "the danger of mercury in fish." For every "good" argument, there was a "bad" argument. The harder she looked for answers, the more confused she became. She started to feel panicky about eating anything!

Amanda had absorbed way too much Food Noise. And it paralyzed her ability to think clearly, tune into her own body's needs, and figure out what was right *for her*.

Food Noise is unavoidable; it's a part of your everyday life. And it's both external and internal. Let's take a look at how you can identify it.

WHAT EXTERNAL FOOD NOISE SOUNDS LIKE

You may not have noticed before, but you're being inundated with Food Noise throughout the day. It shows up in all of the fear-based messages you receive from the media and people around you. This is what it sounds like:

- An advertisement in your favorite magazine telling you to skip breakfast and sip some "metabolism-boosting" detox tea instead.

- An Instagram influencer on day seven of a rigid plan of 100 percent raw vegan food options, no oil, no salt, and absolutely zero processed sugar, ever—and she has a program for you to try, too.

- A conversation on a podcast about a must-try secret ingredient that all the celebrities are raving about.

- An article on Facebook about the "surprising benefits" of a food you've always been taught to avoid.

- A close friend or family member who watched a film about how bad animal protein is for you, and now she's trying to convince you to go vegan as well.

On average, Americans spend more than eleven hours a day consuming media in one form or another. That's almost half a day, every day, being constantly bombarded by messages.[1]

It's no wonder Food Noise can feel so exhausting!

The harm isn't just from listening to all the noise; it's from internalizing it all. Every time those external voices speak up, telling you that you're weak, bad, or not good enough, they crank up the volume on your internal Food Noise.

WHAT INTERNAL FOOD NOISE SOUNDS LIKE

Internal Food Noise has been programmed into your subconscious mind by a lifetime of external Food Noise. And now it pops up in your daily life, disguised as your own thoughts about food. You know the "shoulds," "don'ts," "dos," and accompanying side of guilt?

Internal Food Noise might sound like:

- A dialogue you have with yourself about skipping your boss's birthday celebration with your coworkers because even the thought of cake sets you into a tailspin about how many hours you'll have to spend on the treadmill to burn it off.

- Beating yourself up for eating a cookie after lunch and then telling yourself you're only allowed a big salad for dinner to make up for the cookie.

- Thinking that you need to do a juice cleanse after family pizza night when your jeans feel a little tight the next morning.

- Panicking at the grocery store because they're all out of organic berries and you'd read that conventional produce contains harmful toxins that might cause you to gain weight.

If you've ever thought, "When I lose those last eight pounds, then I deserve to be happy" or "If I'm going out for dinner, I should skip breakfast and lunch," you've fallen victim to Food Noise.

Diet culture is one of the biggest creators of Food Noise, and it's no wonder so many of us falsely buy into its messages. Just think about how often we see images of the "perfect" body! Studies show that children as young as five have concerns about their bodies, and one in four kids have tried dieting by age seven.[2]

That's literally a lifetime of Food Noise in our heads.

THE ROLE OF MODERN DIET CULTURE

Tracking macros, quitting sugar, following a plan, cleansing, detoxing, rebooting, resetting: this is the language of wellness today, and it's intended to make you think "health," not "diet." Because by now we all know that diets don't work, right? The fact is these are all just diets in disguise, and this language is the newest way of sending out the same old Food Noise messages: you're not good enough right now, and there's one "perfect" way you and everyone else should eat.

There is absolutely nothing wrong with trying a trendy superfood or fun workout. Far from it. The only way we learn is by experiencing new things. Otherwise, we become rigid and stuck in our ways. Where the Food Noise gets you is in making you think some new discovery or approach is a miracle cure or that it's necessarily right for you.

Instead, regard a new way of eating or moving with curiosity. Be open. Try it. Take the parts that work for you and ignore the rest. Or decide it's not right for you *at all* and move on, knowing you are not a failure or less than in any way. You are being true to you. No expert, health coach, or fitness instructor knows your body the way you do. They also don't know your circumstances, schedule, and values. Eating dinner at 5 p.m. to fast until the next morning may work for some people, but if your kids don't get home from their afterschool activities until 8 p.m. and that's the only time you have to enjoy a meal together, it may not be right for you.

Quieting the modern diet-culture Food Noise means staying curious and asking yourself: "Where are my actions coming from? Do they feel aligned with my beliefs and what feels good in my body?" If you're feeling out of alignment, then you're just hearing the noise and not what your inner wisdom is trying to tell you.

Tips for Quieting Food Noise

- Limit your exposure to advertisements promoting the latest trend or must-have product. When you're watching TV and commercials come on, use that time to unload the dishwasher, put in a load of laundry, or let the dog out. Can't avoid the ads on social media and in magazines (media makes it hard!)? Remind yourself that what's good for someone else might not work for you. You are the expert of you.

- Avoid food-related chatter. Instead of meeting up for meals or drinks, where there are ample opportunities to generate Food Noise, invite your friend on a hike or take a class together. If they start telling you about a new diet or meal plan, be prepared to gently change the subject. Try something like, "It sounds like you've really put a lot of thought into that. Say, how did [reference a totally different topic that you've talked about in the past] turn out?"

- Flip the script on your internal chatter about food by rewriting your internal Food Noise and tuning into you.

> » Instead of "I should really be eating more
> _____," try "I know myself. I trust myself. I'm
> doing what's right for me."
>
> » Instead of "I read that I shouldn't be eating
> _____," try "I can eat what I like, as long as I
> am honest about how I feel after I eat it."
>
> » Instead of "I don't know what to eat! Food is so
> confusing!" try "I am qualified to listen to my
> body and know what it needs."

FOOD NOISE CAN COME AND GO

Food Noise is sneaky because, while it's what we're hearing *now*, it can also trigger old insecurities or doubts we've worked so hard to overcome.

My client Brooke grew up with a mom who counted and measured every single morsel of food. She would constantly hear her mom assign numbers to all her meals, along with explanations of why she should eat low-fat foods or eliminate fat altogether. Brooke subconsciously absorbed all this information, and food became one big math equation instead of nourishment or, God forbid, pleasure.

It wasn't until Brooke became pregnant in her late twenties that she was able to stop hearing those numbers in her own head and start listening to her body instead. Her pregnancy was smooth, and she felt connected to herself more than ever by eating for nourishment and honoring all her cravings. The Food Noise she'd lived with for so long dissipated, and she could actually enjoy grocery shopping, cooking, and eating!

But after having two kids in three years, Brooke felt overwhelmed by the way her body had changed, and her confidence plummeted. Finding time to work out or even sit down to a real meal seemed nearly impossible. Worse, the other new moms Brooke now spent time with constantly chatted about getting back to their prebaby bodies.

She heard about everything from hard-core, seven-days-a-week, high-intensity exercise classes to surgical tummy tucks to counting macros! All that Food Noise triggered Brooke's old thought patterns, along with a chorus of negative self-talk. She started obsessing about numbers and felt like she was having the same annoying conversations in her head that she had released so long ago.

Finally, she decided to politely change the topics with the other moms when it turned to food and body talk. And with a few of the loudest moms, Brooke even declined playdates altogether. By identifying the Food Noise, Brooke could turn down the volume and think about what she needed to do to feel like herself again. She splurged on a comfortable double stroller to fit both kids—an investment in her new fitness routine. Walking outside wasn't "hard-core," but it felt great to move. She started to feel better and was then inspired to make better choices with food. After just a few days, the Food Noise in her head began to clear.

Just like it did for Brooke, old Food Noise can sometimes reappear when things seem out of control, uncertain, or unstable. And it makes sense, right? When we're stressed or under pressure, it's easier for the noise to seep through and crack the foundation we've so carefully built. This is when it's even more important to be vigilant about quieting the Food Noise. Awareness is key. You have to tune into yourself and pay extra attention to what feels best to you, regardless of how loud the Food Noise becomes.

QUIETING THE NOISE

Just as it's difficult to think clearly when you're inside a chaotic shopping mall, it's difficult to take good care of your body when you're surrounded by loud Food Noise. Uncovering and then eliminating my Food Noise helped me tune back into my own body and identify what it needed to thrive.

I went on to run multiple races after my first marathon. And by allowing myself to listen to my own internal cues, I even exceeded my personal goals and qualified for one of the hardest races in the country, the Boston Marathon.

Crossing the finish line at Boston was one of the best and also one of the most pivotal moments in my life. My biggest lesson? When you quiet the Food Noise and tune into the wisdom of your body, it will tell you *exactly* what it needs in order to feel and do its best.

Worksheet: Eliminate Your Food Noise

Now that you understand Food Noise is unavoidable, whenever you notice Food Noise throughout your day, think to yourself: "Food Noise Alert!" (or "FNA!" for short). Just because Food Noise is everywhere does not mean you are powerless! You can take charge and dial down the volume.

FIND YOUR FOOD NOISE

Walk through your house and look at the books on your shelves. Scroll through your Instagram feed and look at the influencers you follow. Think about the last conversation you had with a friend about food. Try to remember what you last told yourself when you sat down to a meal.

Check off the sources of Food Noise currently present in your life:

- ☐ Instagram and other social media influencers
- ☐ TV, radio, and podcast commercials
- ☐ celebrity gossip tabloids and other magazines
- ☐ blogs and websites
- ☐ e-newsletters
- ☐ friends
- ☐ family
- ☐ diet and nutrition books
- ☐ colleagues
- ☐ other sources of Food Noise: _____

Which Food Noise Alerts did you check off?

For each item you checked off, ask yourself, "What's my plan to erase (or at least minimize) this source of Food Noise?"

Your action steps can be really simple. They can look something like: "Unsubscribe from this newsletter; get rid of those old cleanse books; tell Mom that I love her, but I don't want to talk about her new diet anymore."

Each time you eliminate Food Noise, you're clearing space in your mind and in your life and giving yourself a clean slate to make choices that feel right for and aligned to you.

My plan to eliminate Food Noise:

CHAPTER 7

Don't Bring Stress to the Table

can still taste the chocolate . . .

I'm on the coast of Mexico with my husband celebrating our anniversary. The weather is ideal. The beaches are pristine and beautiful. And then there's the food. Fresh, juicy papaya. Rich, creamy guacamole. Ginger-lime juice. Thick, rustic masa tacos bursting with spice-rubbed local fish. Sweet chili pepper tamales. And the bread! Warm and crusty with pockets of melted chocolate tucked inside. I eat all of it! I mean *all* of it. Being in the moment like this, free of worry and actually enjoying every bite, is a big departure for me, someone who meticulously plans every meal ahead of time.

I left Mexico feeling happy, energized, and *lighter* in every sense of the word. Has this ever happened to you? You go away, eat differently (or more!), and then come home feeling better than ever? How can this be? This is what is known as the vacation paradox. You feel this way because you *relax* when you're away. You've left the Food Noise back home. Your mind is no longer stuck in that stressful soundtrack of "I feel guilty," "Why don't I have any willpower?" and "Is this really organic?" When you eat in a relaxed way (whether you're on vacation or not), your body is more receptive to taking in the experience, *and* you receive the full nutritional benefits of the foods you eat. Why? Because you released some of your daily stress!

STRESS IS A NUTRIENT BLOCKER

That's right. Stress is the ultimate anti-nutrient. If you're stressed out, your mind thundering with Food Noise and limiting beliefs about eating and food, you will be unable to absorb all of the macronutrients, vitamins, and minerals in the food you're eating. You can load up your plate with kale, quinoa, salmon, avocado, and all kinds of other incredibly nutritious food, but if you're in an anxious state of mind when you sit down to eat, then your body will not receive all the nourishment from that meal. What's happening in your mind is just as important as what you're tossing into your grocery cart. Of course, if you're only tossing in packaged, processed, and other low-quality foods, you can't magically relax those foods into nutrient-dense powerhouses. Relaxation *plus* high-quality food choices are the ideal way to go. Your mind and your mouth are connected, and both matter when it comes to rewriting your food story.

Here's how it works: when you feel agitated, worried, or tense while eating, this stressed-out mood actually changes your body's physiology. Quick side note here: You may not *think* you're stressed out at the table, but if you're hearing Food Noise, trust me, you are stressed. This is a low-level stress, but it is still stress. Any guilt, judgment about health, or shame about your choices is perceived as a stressor by the brain and turns on your sympathetic nervous system, triggering your body's stress response, also known as the fight-or-flight mode. To your body, any kind of stress means, "Danger!" which kicks off a series of events to get you primed to deal with it.

What happens? Well, several things. Your sympathetic nervous system directs the body to produce more cortisol, a stress hormone. Your muscles tense. Your heart starts beating fast. Your blood pressure rises. Your blood sugar goes up. Your appetite increases, especially for sugary, high-carb foods. Your thyroid becomes sluggish, meaning your metabolism slows down. Your digestion shuts off. And your immune system is compromised. With all of this going on, especially having a digestive system offline, how can your body process that colorful, nutrient-dense dinner you prepared? In short, it can't, or at least not fully and completely.

When you're stressed, your body is triggered to protect itself, preserve energy, and store more fat, not digest and assimilate the nutrients in food. Plus your senses are impaired, so your food just doesn't taste as good, and you don't experience as much pleasure from your food as when you're relaxed.

Over time, all of this stress doesn't just hamper the digestive system, it can seriously damage it, weakening the lining of your gut, increasing its permeability (commonly referred to as leaky gut), and harming your microbiome, the collection of bacteria that help break down food.

Crazy, right? All that's happening because of those anxious thoughts about food. When most people think of sources of stress, they think of losing a job, financial challenges, an accident or injury, a health concern, or the loss of a loved one. Or more everyday situations like a tight deadline at work or a driver swerving into your lane on the highway. We don't realize that what's going on in our minds—"I'm going to gain weight," "I need to change my body," "I should eat less carbs"—can trigger our stress response, too. Your body reacts with exactly the same cascade of hormonal changes whether it's an event or a thought that sets off the stress response alarm. And to make things worse, it doesn't matter whether your thoughts are true or not. As long as you believe them, then you can create a stress response.

The big takeaway: what you think has a powerful effect on digestion, and your stressful thoughts start a hormonal cascade that impacts your every bite!

MY WAKE-UP CALL

It was the end of 2012. I had been working with clients for a little over two years, helping women cultivate healthier habits. At that point, the focus was mostly on what to eat: more fruits and veggies, less sugar, more fiber. Even though my clients and I were feeling better from these higher-quality food and lifestyle choices, I kept thinking that something was missing, something that could bring more ease, more joy, more freedom.

Then one day I picked up a book called *The Slow Down Diet* by Marc David, founder of the Institute for the Psychology of Eating. Not to be overly dramatic, but it completely blew my mind. My eyes landed on these words: "Eating healthy food is only half of the story of good nutrition. Being in the ideal state to digest and assimilate food is the other half."[1] Ideal state? What was the ideal state? How could I get there? I wanted to know more.

This was a pivotal moment in my food story. I had never even thought about how my state of mind affected my nutrition. Here I was, practically the poster child for health. I was shopping at the farmers' market, cooking at home, and eating seasonal, whole, real foods every day. I made sure to balance my blood sugar with all my meals and snacks. Heck, I was even making my kids homemade chicken nuggets so they could have the healthier versions of foods they loved. I was doing all the "right" things and felt way more flexible and a lot less rigid than I had in the past. To be honest, I thought I was healed.

But I still worried. I beat myself up over little things, like the times I couldn't make everything from scratch, or deviated from the "plan" and then started over again the next Monday, or didn't feed my sons the most nourishing meals possible. And even though I gathered my family around the table to eat, I sat down with my personal soundtrack playing the same tune day after day:

"Is this a balanced meal?"

"Why did I eat so much?"

"How come I always go for seconds?"

"What is the secret to controlling cravings?"

The truth is, I was preoccupied with being an example for my clients and my children and put an enormous amount of pressure on myself to be the pillar of health. I was worrying and questioning every bite. And although my thoughts shifted from achieving an ideal body to eating the cleanest diet imaginable, I was unknowingly putting undue stress on myself despite my good intentions. By bringing stress to the table, I wasn't getting the full value (or enjoyment!) from my meals. It was completely counterproductive to everything I was trying to accomplish. Once this clicked for me, there was no going back. I enrolled in the Institute for the Psychology of Eating to change my food story and learn new ways to help others, too.

Marc David became my mentor, and he helped me do the deep work needed to see how I was getting in my own way, unwittingly placing obstacles in my own path to true and vibrant health. With his support, I came face-to-face with my eating perfectionism and had to unravel the hard truth: my desire to be a shining example was creating stress, and that stress had no place at my table at all. I will never forget when he told me the ultimate goal was to become a relaxed eater. A relaxed eater! I never even knew that I wasn't a relaxed eater. But the more I thought about it, the more I realized how foreign that manner of eating was to me. I had been a relaxed eater only a few times, like when I went to Mexico and ate all that local fresh food and chocolate bread without a stitch of guilt.

But you don't need to go to Mexico or on any vacation to become a relaxed eater. You can start today at your very next meal. If I can do it, so can you!

BECOME A RELAXED EATER

Trust me, I understand that eating in a relaxed state isn't as easy as it sounds. No one quiets all of their Food Noise, sheds all of their limiting beliefs, silences negative self-talk, and learns to slow down in one fell swoop. But I'm asking you to start the process—to move your body toward relaxation at your meals. You'll reap tremendous health benefits, including improved digestion, by flipping the off switch in your sympathetic nervous system and your body's stress response and turning on your parasympathetic nervous system and your body's relaxation response.

Dr. Herbert Benson, a pioneer in mind/body medicine and currently director emeritus at the Benson-Henry Institute for Mind Body Medicine at Massachusetts General Hospital, coined the term *relaxation response* to describe what happens when you activate the parasympathetic nervous system and your body releases hormones and other chemicals to counteract the stress response and return your heart rate, blood pressure, blood sugar, and digestion back to normal. Think of the relaxation response as the opposite of the stress response:

while stress turns off digestion, relaxation turns it back on. We often shorthand this as *rest and digest.*

SYMPATHETIC NERVOUS SYSTEM	PARASYMPATHETIC NERVOUS SYSTEM
turns on stress response	turns on relaxation response
turns off digestion	turns on digestion

Becoming a relaxed eater is the first step toward tuning into your inner wisdom—a direct line to your intuition and all the answers that live inside you. While relaxed, you'll be more aware and present, so you can notice the sensations of your food and how you respond to it. You'll learn to trust those messages and realize that you are, in fact, your own self-expert.

So how do you approach the table in a more relaxed and less stressed way? How do you flip on the parasympathetic nervous system and stimulate the relaxation response? Start by taking a few deep breaths before eating. As simple as it sounds, deep breathing is one of the most effective ways to prompt the relaxation response, slow your heart rate, and center your mind. It works by stimulating your vagus nerve, the main control switch for your parasympathetic nervous system and the rest and digest response. Simply inhale and exhale before your next meal to move away from stress and into relaxation mode.

Next, I like adding a mantra to create a complete pre-meal ritual. You've probably heard the term *mantra* before. A mantra is a word, phrase, or sound that helps you quiet the noise inside your mind, clear distractions, feel calmer, and concentrate fully on whatever activity you're doing—whether that's meditating, writing, cooking, eating, or anything else. A mantra can be one word (for instance, "focus," "love," "peace," "presence"), a short phrase ("I am safe," "Be here now," "I choose to love myself"), or a sacred sound (in yoga traditions, chanting "Om" is a good example of this).

You may think this all sounds pretty woo-woo, but mantras really do shift your mental state, and there's evidence to back this up. One study from Linköping University in Sweden found that using a mantra "suppresses your brain's default mode network," which is a scientific way of saying that mantras quiet your busy mind. After repeating a mantra, there's a noticeable change in your brain activity.[2] Even better: choose a positive phrase as a mantra ("I am growing stronger every day"), and you get the added benefits of creating new, positive neural pathways to support your new way of thinking while calming your mind. If the word *mantra* doesn't feel good to you, call this positive intention something else: an affirmation, reminder, statement, or pre-meal ritual. Whatever you call it, the effects will be the same.

By taking a few deep breaths and repeating a mantra or other empowering word or phrase to yourself a few times, you'll clear stress from the table, get your brain into an optimal state for your meal, and have a more nourishing experience.

It only takes a few words and a few seconds.

Activity: Use A Mantra Before Your Next Meal

Before your next meal, try using a mantra to relax your body and mind.

Choose your mantra. Your pre-meal mantra can be anything you want. Consider one of these phrases or create another one that resonates with you.

"I am nourishing myself."

"I am savoring this moment."

"It feels good to eat slowly."

"It feels good to take care of myself."

"I am grateful for this meal."

"Thank you, food. Thank you, body."

"Guilt, you are not invited to the table."

"Perfectionism, you are not welcome here."

"My only job right now is to savor this meal."

"Eating can be simple."

"Quiet mind, peaceful meal."

"I am investing in my health."

"I am learning to eat in a new way."

"This is my new food story."

Just before you start eating, take a few deep breaths. Then repeat your chosen mantra to yourself.

You can say your mantra silently (inside your head) or out loud. You'll receive the mental benefits either way.

You can say your mantra once, but for best results, I'd recommend that you repeat it a few times in a row.

After your meal, take a few moments to journal about the experience. How do you feel? Did you find your meal more enjoyable? Do you feel any differently now, after eating with a pre-meal mantra, than you do after eating without one?

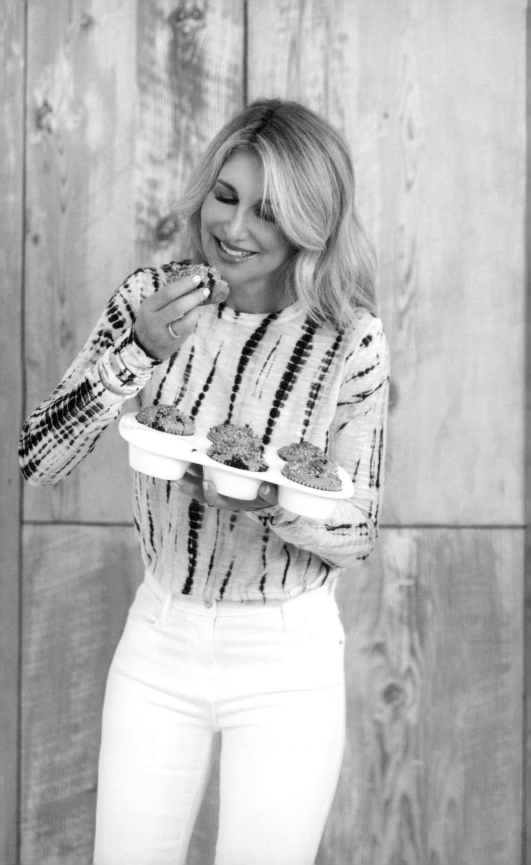

Part 3

RECONNECT WITH YOUR BODY

CHAPTER 8

Invite Yourself to Dinner

magine this: You've had a really stressful week. Friday comes around, and all you can think about is eating a good meal and relaxing. You invite your best friend, Olivia, to come hang with you for dinner. With a fridge filled with fresh ingredients, you're inspired to make a new recipe and cannot wait to enjoy it over a bottle of rosé.

You crank up the tunes and start sautéing the veggies. Soon, your kitchen smells like a Michelin-starred restaurant. Olivia arrives, and as you sit down, you notice that she is totally distracted. She's been looking at her phone since she walked in the door. How rude! She asks you to repeat what you just said multiple times because she's not really listening. And then, she just stares at the food. You know exactly what's going on. She's busy running the numbers in her mind, calculating the carbs and fat grams and obsessing over the macros before even taking a bite. With a resting bitch face, she hesitantly picks up her fork, and you can't help but wonder: is she *actually* going to taste your Genius Guacamole with Toasted Seeds (page 221)?

Somewhere between the Can't Be Beet Burgers (page 211) and the Chocolate-Pistachio Bark with Freeze-Dried Raspberries (page 222), you decide that you aren't going to ask Olivia to come over for a meal again. Ever! You don't want to dine with someone who is unable to give you the gift of presence or appreciate a plate of home-cooked food made with love.

Now, take a moment and consider *your* behavior during meals, both alone and shared with others. How many times have you been on your phone, watching the news, responding to emails, leafing through a magazine, or consumed with thoughts that kept you from fully being a part of the eating experience? Think about all the times that *you have been Olivia.* We all have! Of course, you're not intentionally trying to be distracted while eating. But Olivia is holding up a mirror for us and letting us peek into the reality of what it feels like when we're not *all there* during meals.

I spent at least two decades either living in my head while eating or looking for distractions in order to avoid confronting my feelings around food. We now know that having anxious thoughts about food raises cortisol levels and, conversely, being relaxed at the table allows the body to rest and digest. But maximizing the nourishment you receive from your food is only one benefit to consider. Here's another: satisfaction. It is impossible to be tuned into how food makes you feel—and to actually derive pleasure from it—when you're distracted while eating.

EAT WITHOUT (EXTERNAL AND INTERNAL) DISTRACTIONS

We are a culture of distracted eaters. A 2019 study revealed that 88 percent of the adults polled stare at a screen while eating.[1] Another found that one in three Americans can't eat without their phones on, and 72 percent often watch television while eating.[2] Screens aren't the only distractions. In addition to these external sources, we're often distracted by internal sources, such as a racing mind whirling with obsessive thoughts about food (FNA!) and a never-ending to-do list.

The nonstop demands on our time are often why we fall into the habit of trying to multitask while eating. It's easy to feel as if eating and multitasking go hand in hand—you can eat while doing almost anything. You can grab your smoothie while you're running out the door. You can send out emails *while* you're shoveling in lunch. You can watch that new Netflix series *while* you're sitting down to dinner. You can plan out your workouts to burn off your meal *while* munching on your 3 p.m. snack. We pride ourselves on being able to do two things at once and "get things done."

But multitasking is a myth. It has been scientifically proven that multitasking doesn't save time. In fact, you lose time, because the brain cannot effectively or efficiently switch between tasks.[3] Studies have shown that we are more likely to forget some of the tasks we're trying to juggle and make more errors when multitasking.[4] Have you ever stared at the bottom of an empty hummus container *while* scrolling through social media and wondered how the heck you managed to finish that last bite? (My hand is raised, too.)

Multitasking makes it impossible to eat in the moment. If you're preoccupied and busy, you can't possibly listen carefully to your body's needs and wants. At the very least, you aren't tuned into your hunger and fullness cues, but the problem goes beyond that, too. You miss all the little nuances that might arise, such as whether a food agrees with you physically or how it makes you feel emotionally. Bottom line: you simply can't tune into your senses and derive satisfaction from your food when your attention is diluted and spread thin. And you deserve to! You deserve to enjoy and savor the meals you spend time preparing or that someone prepares for you. You're worthy of taking a few minutes to put yourself into a relaxed state, free of distractions, before taking the first bite, even if you're dining by yourself.

You might be thinking, "But I don't have time to eat in the moment!" Let me assure you: you *can* eat in the moment—even if you're overwhelmingly busy, even if you don't have a lot of time. I want to emphasize that eating without distractions doesn't necessarily mean you're lounging around, nibbling chilled fruit for hours (although that does sound luxurious!). Eating in the moment is about the *intentionality* you bring to the meal, not the actual duration of it. Whether you take five minutes or a full hour to eat your lunch, you're choosing to be fully present during that time.

So it's time to invite yourself to dinner and take a seat at the table. Put away your phone and laptop, turn off the TV, and clear your mind of any extra chatter. If you're dining with someone, give that person your undivided attention. Think of it as single-tasking! I can tell you from firsthand experience that this is a much better way to approach mealtime, fostering a deeper connection to your food and the people around you and nourishing you in a soul-satisfying way.

Crystal came to me with one request: "I want to be able to listen to my body." She found this nearly impossible to do with all the noise and busyness that took over every time she sat down to eat. She told me that she almost always felt "stuffed" after her meals and that she hardly ever enjoyed them, with all the negative self-talk going on inside her head.

First, Crystal needed to stop bringing her stress to the table. I asked Crystal if she would be willing to spend one minute before eating to get into a better mindset. I gave her the option of reciting a mantra (refer back to the exercise in chapter 7 for a refresher), taking a few deep breaths, or thinking about what she appreciated about her day. Any one of these options would help Crystal turn on her parasympathetic nervous system, create awareness of her actions and thoughts, and become a more relaxed eater. Moving from ungrounded and stressed to grounded and relaxed before she ate would bring her into the magic of the moment.

Crystal opted to take a few deep breaths before sitting down for a meal and found this simple exercise served as a barrier to the stress she was feeling. Now that Crystal was in the present moment, her next step was to stay there, resisting any urge to let her mind wander. It took practice! But Crystal quickly noticed how much more flavorful her food tasted and how she could more easily *hear* her body telling her when it was full. She paid attention to the little nuances that she had missed out on all this time. Without distractions, Crystal was able to finally connect to her inner wisdom, stop eating when she felt satisfied, and avoid feeling unpleasantly overstuffed.

Three Steps to Getting Connected

1. Encourage the relaxation response prior to your meal. Use your mantra or take a few deep breaths.

2. Once you are eating, stay in the present moment. Resist the urge to pick up your phone or let your mind wander.

3. Tune into the nuances of the meal and your inner wisdom.

Like Crystal, you can start to feel connected to your food and body, too. Once you elicit your relaxation response and are in a calm state, present in the moment, get comfortable staying there. Resist the temptation to reply to a text or rerun an earlier conversation with your boss. Notice your meal. The colors. The smells. The anticipation of eating it. The way it makes you feel with that very first bite. How present you are with the experience. How much more tuned in you are with yourself and, if you're not alone, with others as well.

When you replace distraction with connection, you open yourself up to experiencing that connection—to your food, your body, and your loved ones—in many different ways. You can feel connected to your food by appreciating how it was grown and where it came from. You can feel connected to the process of making a beautiful meal and enjoy the details of the preparation. You can feel connected to the subtle sensations created by your mind and body as they respond to each bite. You can feel connected to the pleasure you're experiencing as you eat or the comfort of a satisfied belly after you're all done. You can feel connected to the conversation with your friends or family sitting at the table. You can feel all sorts of connections that nourish your mind, body, and soul on a deep level. But none of them can happen until you give yourself (and others) your undivided focus and attention.

Ready to experience all of the benefits of connection? Forget waiting until your next meal to start! Let's take a few minutes right now to turn away from distractions and tune into the moment. And did I mention chocolate is involved?

Activity: The Chocolate Meditation

Meditation is an incredibly powerful way to quiet your mind and tune into your senses in the present moment. It offers so many emotional and physical benefits: your sympathetic nervous system settles down, your stress levels drop, and your cognitive function improves (translation: you're able to think more clearly). If you've never meditated before or think there's no way it's for you, please hang with me for just a moment. The truth is, I'm not very good at meditating . . . but add some chocolate? Totally different story! Give this guided Chocolate Meditation a try, and I think you'll be pleasantly surprised at the experience.

The point of doing this exaggerated exercise is to illustrate the power of presence in your food story and help you understand what it means to connect to your food and feel completely satisfied, too. You'll close your eyes and savor a piece of dark chocolate. You'll practice slowing down, eating in the moment, and engaging all of your senses to experience chocolate in a whole new way, tuning into all the little details that you miss when you're not 100 percent present with your food. I have led thousands of people through this short exercise, and almost everyone is blown away by the difference that bringing every sense to the table can make. Once you experience it, you will understand why one of the participants, a jolly guy named Joe, came up to me two weeks later and said, "I can still taste the chocolate."

You will need:

- A few small pieces of chocolate—ideally, high-quality dark chocolate.

- A comfortable place to sit: on the floor, on the couch, on a chair at a table or desk, anywhere!

Let's begin. Make sure that you are sitting comfortably. Close your eyes and take a few deep, slow breaths. Notice how just the simple act of breathing deeply already creates a change in how you feel. Bring your mind to be here now, not worrying about what happened earlier in the day or what you need to do later. By keeping your mind in the present moment, you'll get the greatest benefits from this meditation.

Keep breathing slowly and deeply. Feel the ground or the furniture beneath you. Feel the connection to and support of the earth. Notice the sounds around you. First, try to listen for a sound that's very far away. Maybe a distant car horn. Or children playing outside. Notice that distant sound.

Next, see if you can notice a sound that's much closer. Maybe a sound right inside your room. The hum of the refrigerator. The sound of rain on your roof. Your dog snoring quietly in the corner. A sound very close to you. Notice that sound.

And then, notice the sound of your own breath. You might hear a faint sound through your nose, your mouth. Notice your own inhaling and exhaling. Bring your awareness inward. Take a moment to just be here, right now. Release the to-do lists or other racing thoughts in your mind.

Slowly, staying in this very relaxed place, notice the chocolate that's in front of you. Pick it up and feel its weight in your hand. Observe its shape and color. Touch and feel its texture between your fingertips as you pick it up. Silently describe the chocolate to yourself: is it dark, smooth, square?

Bring the chocolate up to your nose and inhale deeply. Follow the scent as it travels into your nose and to the back of your nostrils. Inhale and exhale deeply for a few moments. Be aware of what is happening in your mind. Are you anticipating eating the chocolate? Does it have more of an aroma than you realized?

Place the chocolate in your mouth. As you begin to chew slowly, observe any burst of flavor, subtle or strong. Hold the chocolate in your mouth for as long as possible, exploring the taste, the textures, and all the subtleties that you might not usually notice.

Roll the chocolate around against the roof of your mouth. Be aware of any feelings, sensations, or memories of your first bite of chocolate. Maybe it was a Hershey's Kiss or a bar with crunchy, sweet almonds.

Even as you're still eating this piece of chocolate, you might feel a desire to quickly reach for another. See if you can relax and stay focused on what you are experiencing in this moment rather than jumping forward and anticipating that next bit of flavor. Keep experiencing the chocolate, slowly savoring each bite.

Finally, when the chocolate is gone, bring your attention back to your senses. Notice whether there is still a residual taste in your mouth. Close your eyes once more and take deep breaths in and out.

Enjoy any difference you feel in your body and mind. Think about how in just a few minutes you were able to quiet your mind, tune into your senses, and feel what was happening in the moment.

Your Chocolate Meditation is now complete! Hopefully, this experiment gave you a little glimpse into the benefits of tuning into your body, engaging your senses, and being fully present with your food. Most people tell me that they can't believe how much better everything tastes when they eat this way. Take another few minutes to write down some of your observations. How do you feel? What did you notice?

\
\
\
\
\
\
\

Remember: this Chocolate Meditation is an exaggerated exercise to illustrate the power of presence in your food story. Of course, it's not realistic to eat every single meal so slowly and with such undivided attention or to have it drag on for hours. However, it is possible to stay connected while eating by minimizing distractions for five, ten, or twenty minutes. And when you give yourself (and others) the gift of presence, you'll soon realize how incredible it feels for you and everyone around you, too. By opening the door and becoming present in one area of your life, you magically unlock the power to become present in all areas of your life.

CHAPTER 9

Use Food to Boost your Mood

The room was packed with eager people coming to hear my sold-out talk, "A Food for Every Mood." Both excited and nervous to share this cutting-edge information, I began by asking a few questions.

"How many of you have ever eaten something and felt totally off? Uncomfortable? Unfocused?

"Raise your hand if you've ever felt anxious about food. You've worried, 'Is this gonna go straight to my thighs?' or 'If I eat this, am I going to feel bloated and regret it later?'

"And raise your hand if you sometimes feel bored or stuck with food—like, you don't know what to make for dinner. You just don't feel excited to get in the kitchen. ME TOO!"

I had their attention. I continued, "Today, I'm going to help you feel less stressed about food. Because food should not be stressful! Food should be nourishing, pleasurable, and joyful. Instead of feeling anxious about food, I want you to feel *inspired and empowered*. Would you like to feel inspired and empowered?" A sea of heads nodded yes in unison.

You could practically hear a pin drop as I shared with them what I'm about to share with you: a new, revitalizing way to think about food.

One that unsticks you from old habits and old stories while injecting a healthy dose of fun. One that reenergizes the way you eat the rainbow and enjoy lots and lots of nutrient-dense, fiber-rich, blood-sugar-balancing foods. One that offers you a way to support your mood so you feel great all day.

Meet the *food-mood connection*, one of the most exciting, transformative, and science-backed ways to think about food. It offers up a proactive approach to eating that changes the narrative inside your mind. It works like this: instead of worrying about what food can do *to* you, you start thinking about everything it can do *for* you. Even though that might sound subtle, it makes all the difference. Are you ready to flip the script?

A NEW WAY TO THINK ABOUT FOOD

I'm guessing you've already noticed some of the ways food can influence your mood. Perhaps you've found that foods rich in tryptophan, such as turkey, eggs, flax, and honey, make you feel cozy or even sleepy. Or possibly you've realized that sugar and caffeine give you a burst of energy and drive, followed by an awful crash that leaves you sluggish and depleted. Or maybe you have even seen products with names like "Bliss," with ingredients such as cacao and mushroom adaptogens (a select group of super mushrooms that adapt to what your body needs and naturally help counteract stress) to promote calm, or "Glow," made with turmeric, ginger, ashwagandha, and other supportive ingredients to help you feel brighter and more refreshed. That's the food-mood connection.

Most of us are intuitively aware of the ways food impacts how we feel and that when we eat real, whole foods, we feel better than when we eat junk foods. Science is catching up to our intuition, confirming that certain foods, such as fruits, nuts, seeds, and healthy fats, can help us feel motivated and upbeat while others, such as processed foods and refined sugar, can dampen our spirits. This doesn't mean those cheesy puffs are evil or that you should never have them. (Remember: there is no such thing as "good" or "bad" food anyway.) It's just helpful to be aware of how these foods make you feel, so you can make empowered choices throughout the day.

And right there is how the food-mood connection can transform the way you think about food. It puts the power of choice in your hands!

It works like this: you choose a specific mood—an emotional state, a feeling—that you want to experience, and then you select ingredients that promote this exact mood. For instance, if you want to feel calm, you can enjoy some dark chocolate. It boosts anandamide, known as the bliss molecule, which helps you to calm down and bliss out.[1]

Or maybe you don't want to feel super calm right now. You have a tight deadline at work and need to ramp up your focus and concentration. The brain-boosting healthy fats in an avocado or walnuts are just what you need to help you think more clearly and feel sharper.

Of course, you'll experience the benefits of mood-boosting foods only if you're in the right frame of mind. Mindset matters, remember? When you're agitated, worried, tense, or continuously hearing Food Noise during a meal, your stressed-out mood actually changes your body's physiology. So even if you're eating something really nutrient dense, such as a Mediterranean Collard Wraps with a romesco sauce (page 235), you're not getting the full benefits of that nourishing dish. And why, when you're in a relaxed mood, you reap maximum nourishment from your food.

Now that you're getting good at tuning into the emotions and behaviors you're bringing to the table, you're ready to start turning your attention to the specific science-backed mood-boosting benefits food can bring you.

THE FOOD-MOOD CONNECTION IS REAL

The connection between food and mood is an emerging field in science. A lot of research is being done to figure out exactly how it all works, but there's no mistaking the link. Many studies over the past several years have confirmed the power of food to impact our state of mind. For example:

- A 2011 study published in the *American Journal of Clinical Nutrition* found that women who ate more vitamin D–rich foods were happier and enjoyed life more.[2]

- Researchers have found that people who eat a Mediterranean diet show improved cognitive function, especially better memory and attention.[3]

- A nine-year study following nearly three hundred people found that eating more fruits and vegetables lowers the risk of both depression and anxiety.[4]

- Frequent consumption of fermented foods packed with probiotics, the live bacteria that support a healthy gut microbiome, alleviates anxiety and promotes a happier outlook overall.[5]

This is just a taste of the findings. New research is being released all of the time. If this still sounds too good to be true, it won't once you get a handle on how your body works.

Your brain produces chemical messengers called *neurotransmitters*, which carry signals that influence a variety of functions throughout your body, such as heart rate, sleep, appetite, and mood. Key neurotransmitters that play a role in mood include:

- Serotonin: helps you feel upbeat, calm, and more focused, which is why it's often referred to as the "happy chemical."

- Dopamine: plays a role in reward and motivation, and a large amount creates feelings of pleasure or emotional "highs."

- Gamma-aminobutyric acid (GABA): regulates anxiety and supports feelings of relaxation and calm.

We can harness the power of neurotransmitters to influence mood by eating foods that boost their production or make it easier for them to do their job.

Mood is influenced in large part by neurotransmitters, so eating to support them is a major way to regulate it, but not the only way. A healthy body promotes a healthy mood. Choosing foods containing nutrients that keep your body humming in all sorts of essential ways, such as by clearing toxins, lowering inflammation, and boosting the immune system, is another way to optimize your physical and emotional well-being.

And we can't forget about the role of gut-healing foods. Your gut is directly connected to your brain and mood—so much so it's actually been called "the second brain." An estimated 90 percent (or more!) of the feel-good neurotransmitter serotonin is manufactured in your gut.

A balanced gut microbiome with plenty of "good" bacteria is key for producing serotonin. Alternatively, poor gut health is associated with chronic inflammation throughout the body, which is in turn overwhelmingly associated with mood swings, anxiety, and depression.[6] When you improve your gastrointestinal health, you simultaneously improve your mental health, too.

So what are some of these specific mood-boosting nutrients? Look no further than your pantry and refrigerator.

PROTEIN: Amino acids, the building blocks of protein, are needed to make neurotransmitters. Tryptophan, an amino acid found in fish, eggs, chicken, turkey, peanuts, pumpkin seeds, sesame seeds, and other proteins, is necessary for the creation of serotonin. We need the tyrosine in almonds, avocados, and dairy products to make dopamine. The main component of GABA is the amino acid glutamine, found in legumes, brown rice, and spinach.

HEALTHY FATS: With about 60 percent of your brain made of fat, it's no wonder that good-for-you fats, especially those rich in omega-3 fatty acids, are crucial for optimal brain function and mood, improving neurotransmitter activity and lowering inflammation. Sources include walnuts, flaxseeds, avocados, and salmon.

COMPLEX CARBOHYDRATES: Whole grains, legumes, fruits, and vegetables provide important nutrients and fiber while clearing the way for tryptophan to easily enter your brain and boost your serotonin levels. That's why not getting enough complex carbs can have a negative impact on your mood. And yes, you read that right. Grains and beans aren't your only option. Fruits and both starchy and non-starchy vegetables are excellent sources of complex carbs!

B VITAMINS: Capable of increasing levels of serotonin, dopamine, and GABA and improving their signaling power, B vitamins are a superstar feel-good nutrient.[7] Salmon, leafy greens, and legumes are packed with a variety of B vitamins.

MAGNESIUM: Found in dark chocolate, avocados, nuts, seeds, legumes, leafy greens, and whole grains, the anti-stress mineral regulates GABA, helping you to release tension and relax. Magnesium is involved in more than three hundred chemical reactions in the body, and some studies suggest more than 75 percent of Americans don't meet their daily requirement.[8] Luckily, there are an abundance of magnesium-rich foods to choose from.

ANTIOXIDANTS: Free radicals—compounds that over time can cause harm to your body, including your nervous system, and have been linked to depression and anxiety—are constantly being formed in your body. Antioxidants keep them in check. Berries, bursting with antioxidant flavonoids, have been shown to boost brain health, mood, and memory. Researchers at Harvard's Brigham and Women's Hospital found that women who consumed two or more servings of strawberries and blueberries each week delayed memory decline by up to two and a half years.[9] And bring on the kale, collards, and spinach! Leafy greens are loaded with antioxidants to keep your mind clear and focused.

ANTI-INFLAMMATORIES: Inflammation throughout your body means inflammation in your brain and your gut, compromising their ability to function and sabotaging your mood. Anti-inflammatory foods keep inflammation in check and boost your immunity. Berries, oranges, lemons, limes, and bell peppers are packed with vitamin C, a potent anti-inflammatory, while carrots and sweet potatoes are stocked with beta carotene, which your body converts to vitamin A, another nutritional powerhouse. Bold spices such as turmeric, ginger, garlic, cinnamon, cloves, oregano, thyme, and rosemary can help reduce inflammation while enhancing flavor, memory, and focus.

PROBIOTICS: Live microorganisms support the healthy bacteria in your gut and may even raise serotonin levels. Reach for fermented foods such as kimchi, yogurt (dairy and non-dairy), kefir, kombucha, miso, or sauerkraut.

FIBER: Healthy gut bacteria love plant fiber, especially inulin, a type of prebiotic (or food for probiotics) naturally found in leeks, garlic, onions, artichokes, asparagus, lentils, slightly green bananas, and oats. Fiber also helps to keep your blood sugar stable, preventing those rollercoaster spikes and crashes throughout the day and the mood swings and irritability that go along with them.

See how food is really your friend? After all those years of worrying what a meal might do *to* you, keep reminding yourself of all the incredible things it does *for* you. It can give you energy, promote a positive outlook, enhance your brain power, regulate hormones, and simply bring you pleasure. You can proactively choose foods based on your desired mood.

SO HOW DO YOU WANT TO FEEL?

My all-time favorite question to ask my clients, my community, and myself is: "How do you want to feel?" Don't be surprised if I encourage you to ask yourself this question a lot throughout this book. Why? Because checking in with yourself regularly can help you determine whether how you want to feel and how you *are* feeling are aligned. And if not, it can help you figure out how to get them in sync. Food is one possible way to go.

You want to feel focused? Happy? Comforted? Sensual? Let's start pinpointing some specific foods to support those states! I've found that most of us are looking to encourage one of the following seven moods.

Happy

To feel happy (uplifted, elevated, cheerful, optimistic) choose:

- Vibrant, colorful foods (red beets, orange pumpkins, yellow curries, green veggies, blue and purple berries), which are nutritious and visually stimulating, too.

- Legumes (chickpeas, lentils, peas, beans) to support and boost production of the happiness neurotransmitter serotonin.

- Healthy fats (avocado, nuts, fish), especially foods rich in omega-3 fatty acids (chia, flax, hemp), which can help stave off depression.

- Foods that provide L-theanine, an amino acid that can help you feel calm, less irritable, and happier overall (matcha tea, cacao).

- Good sources of B vitamins (Brazil nuts, dark, leafy greens, whole grains) to lift your spirits.

Focused

To feel focused (sharp, clear, awake, alert) choose:

- Healthy fats (avocado, nuts, fish) to keep your brain—which is 60 percent fat—functioning optimally.

- Greens (kale, spinach, collards, broccoli), which are packed with brain-boosting nutrients such as vitamin K, lutein, folate, and beta carotene.

- Anti-inflammatory spices (garlic, turmeric, ginger, cinnamon, cloves, oregano, thyme, rosemary) to help reduce tension-related headaches.

- Good sources of magnesium (hemp seeds, cashews, almonds, quinoa, high-quality dark chocolate) to enjoy the benefits of the anti-stress mineral.

- Probiotics and fermented foods for a healthy gut and a healthy brain, too.

- Balanced meals with a mix of macronutrients (protein, carbs, and fat) each time you eat so you feel satiated and energized.

- Regular meals so your blood sugar never gets too low, because it's hard to focus when you're hangry!

Radiant

To feel radiant (glowing, gorgeous, bright, vibrant) choose:

- Foods rich in vitamin C (brightly colored fruits and vegetables like pomegranates, citrus fruits, and yellow peppers) to boost collagen production and produce firm, healthy skin and a strong heart.

- Protein (chickpeas, beans, lentils, salmon, tuna, chicken, edamame, veggie burgers, eggs), another crucial ingredient for collagen production.

- Plenty of water, because dehydration leaves you feeling tired, dry, and dull, both physically and emotionally. Drink lots of pure water and also consider soothing teas, homemade broth, and juicy fruits like watermelon.

- Anti-inflammatory spices (garlic, turmeric, ginger, cinnamon, cloves, oregano, thyme, rosemary) to prevent puffy skin.

- Foods high in beta carotene (carrots and sweet potatoes), which your body converts into vitamin A, for gorgeous skin.

Strong

To feel strong (powerful, vital, healthy, unstoppable, immune) choose:

- Beverages and elixirs to strengthen your immune system and help fight off cold and flu bugs. Try hot water with lemon, ginger, and raw honey, and for an extra boost add extract of elderberry, an antiviral.

- A nutrient-dense anti-inflammatory juice or smoothie (turmeric, ginger, cilantro, pineapple, and leafy greens) to boost your immune system even more.

- Probiotic-rich foods (fermented vegetables, miso, yogurt, and sauerkraut) for a healthy gut and strong immune system.

- Foods packed with L-theanine (matcha tea, cacao), a mood-boosting, stress-reducing amino acid that leaves you feeling strong but without the jittery spike and crash of caffeine.

Comforted
To feel comforted (snuggly, relaxed, supported, nostalgic) choose:

- Foods containing tryptophan (salmon, chicken, turkey, eggs, flaxseed, sesame seeds, pumpkin seeds, sunflower seeds, cashews, peanuts, almonds, walnuts, and honey), an amino acid that alleviates anxiety and promotes deep sleep.

- Foods high in potassium (bananas, oranges, cantaloupe, honeydew melons, apricots, spinach, sweet potatoes) and magnesium (spinach, quinoa, nuts, avocados), both of which are natural muscle relaxants to help get those cozy vibes flowing.

- Warm, comforting meals and drinks. One study from Yale University found that holding a warm cup of coffee—rather than iced coffee—changed people's emotional state, making them feel more connected to others and more generous.[10]

- Foods cooked over an open fire! A grill, a barbecue, a campfire. Research shows that being near crackling flames lowers blood pressure and puts people into a deeply relaxed, trancelike state.[11]

- Meals that feel nostalgic and bring back fond memories for you. Sometimes you need the real deal, but other times an updated, healthier version is just as satisfying—like Homemade Nut Butter and Raspberry Chia Jam on Toasts (page 256), a grown-up PB and J.

Sensual
To feel sensual (sexy, confident, relaxed, open, liberated) choose:

- Foods with aphrodisiac properties (dark chocolate, oysters, figs, apples, strawberries, avocados).

- Watermelon and pomegranate juice, good sources of citrulline, a vasodilator, which means it dilates blood vessels.

- Maca powder, made from Peruvian ginseng, which boosts libido and energy levels. Try a teaspoon in your smoothie.

- Foods rich in zinc (pumpkin seeds, pine nuts, chickpeas, lentils, beans, whole grains) to help support the body's production of sex hormones, such as testosterone and prolactin.

- Foods that evoke sensual, sexy memories and feelings: a drizzle of honey, deep red raspberries, chilled grapes, or homemade plant-based truffles made with dates, almond butter, and dark chocolate.

Calm

To feel calm (steady, grounded, centered, chill, blissed out, relaxed) choose:

- Selenium-rich foods (Brazil nuts, yellowfin tuna, mushrooms, lentils). Selenium has been linked to a decrease in anxiety levels and and an improvement in moods.[12]

- Dark chocolate, which contains anandamide, a fatty acid neurotransmitter known as the bliss molecule. Another source of anandamide? Black truffles.

- Chamomile tea, as several studies have shown this flower's power to provide anxiety relief.[13]

- Turmeric, which contains curcumin, a compound that supports brain health and helps alleviate stress.

- Saffron, nicknamed the "sunshine spice," which has been found to brighten your mood and may even reduce symptoms of PMS.[14]

- CBD, derived from the cannabis plant. Unlike THC, which causes you to feel high or stoned, CBD does not have any psychotropic effects. It creates a very subtle, calming, chill-out effect, much like chamomile tea. CBD is available in many forms: as a pure oil that you can add to recipes or infused into chocolate, honey, and other foods.

Keep asking yourself: How do I want to feel? Use the suggestions above and the Food-Mood Cheat Sheets in the "Recipes and Rituals" section for lists of foods and spices to promote your desired mood.

Not sure how to combine these colorful, nutrient-dense foods and spices into your meals? I got you covered! All the recipes in this book are organized by mood. So once you decide how you want to feel, you can cook and eat accordingly!

FEEL EMPOWERED

Are you feeling empowered yet? I hope so! The food-mood connection offers you an opportunity to turn the page on an old, disempowering food story and take charge, plan ahead, and make nourishing choices that steer your mood, your day, and your life in the direction you want. You can be proactive rather than reactive. This is exciting!

Before eating, check in and ask yourself, "How do I want to feel? What could I choose that will help me feel that way?" Use your answers to guide your food choices. Asking yourself that essential question puts you in the driver's seat. With food as your friend, banish hopelessness and overwhelm and step into your power!

Activity: A Food-Mood Journaling Exercise

Use this journaling exercise to help you tune in and notice the connection between what you eat and how you feel. Not in a reactive way ("Ugh, I ate ___, and now I don't feel good!") but, rather, in a proactive way ("I want to feel ___, so I'm going to eat ___ to help generate that mood").

MORNING: PLANNING

How do you want to feel today?

Write down a few words to describe the feelings/emotions/mood you want to experience today. For instance: happy, focused, radiant, strong, comforted, sensual, calm, etc.

What's your plan? How will you create the mood that you want?

What could you eat/drink today to generate the mood you want? If you're not sure, refer to the Food-Mood Cheat Sheets or look at some food-mood recipes. Write down some ideas.

How did your day go? Did you experience the feelings/emotions/mood that you were hoping for?

Did you eat anything today that felt really great for your body and mind? Write down what you noticed.

Did you eat anything today that didn't feel so good for you? Anything that made you feel bloated, itchy, inflamed, sluggish, uncomfortable, or just off in some way? Write down what you noticed.

It's always beautiful to end your day on a positive note. What mood-boosting food are you excited to try next?

CHAPTER 10

How Do You Want to Feel?

am just tired of myself," Heather told me wearily during our first
meeting, literally slumped over in her chair.

"When you say you feel tired," I asked, "what do you mean?" I
invited her to dig a little deeper. Heather was tired of feeling stressed
out about food. She was exhausted from worrying about calories, carbs,
and portion sizes. She was worn out from feeling guilty whenever she
ate something that deviated from "the plan." Heather was constantly
preoccupied with obsessing over which foods were okay to eat and how
much she was allowed to eat and when. Trying to follow so many rules
around food was draining and depleting her energy. Heather told me
about her typical breakfast (a small cup of yogurt) and lunch (low-calorie
bread, turkey slices, one apple) and how tedious and boring it all felt.

"But it's not just the food stuff," she explained. "I just feel *tired*. Peri-
od." Heather went on about the breakneck pace of her life, her packed
calendar, the inbox overflowing with unread messages, and the perpet-
ual feeling that she was giving more than she was receiving. Heather
has two children whom she adores with every fiber of her being. But
the seemingly endless demands of each child made her feel like she had
two additional full-time jobs.

I asked Heather, "When you think about food and your whole life, how would you like to feel?"

"Less tired. Less stressed. Calmer. Happier. More energized. I was hoping that you could tell me exactly what to eat to help me with all of this."

Of course, I had ideas on how Heather could use food to boost her mood, focusing on specific nutrients to help her feel calmer and happier. It was a good place to begin to change how Heather was showing up in her life. But it was just that—a beginning.

THINK BEYOND THE PLATE

There is no doubt about it: what you eat impacts how you feel. Food is an incredibly powerful tool in your mood-boosting toolbox, and it has almost immediate effects. But don't stop there! How you feel about food, your job, family, exercise, and your whole life, really, is a direct reflection of *all* of the daily decisions you make.

Yes, you are making dozens and dozens of food choices every single day, but consider how you can go *beyond the plate* and double down on all of the other ways you can proactively support your mood. This may mean changing things up with your lifestyle in some pretty unexpected ways. I mean, you can eat for happiness all you want, but you won't feel better at work if you stay stuck in a soul-sucking job. The good news is that mood-boosting foods will nourish your body and brain as you navigate these situations, giving you the strength and energy to do so.

Once all of your choices, on and off the plate, are working together, mood support will feel effortless. And you'll feel awesome, because what you're eating and what you're doing are in alignment. Everything is in sync.

During that first conversation with Heather, I asked her the million-dollar question that I ask all of my clients: "Are you willing to try some new things, including new things that aren't even about food?"

Heather agreed that she was willing—but with one important exception.

"Don't you dare take away my three o'clock whipped caramel latte," she said.

Every day at three o'clock, Heather would go to her neighborhood cafe and order a blended coffee drink with her custom-tailored modifications: skim milk, light whip, three shots of espresso, a dash of caramel. She told me she "needed" this drink every day. I asked her why.

"Well, the kids get home at three thirty," she explained.

"And when the kids get home, then what happens?" I asked. "How does that feel?"

Heather paused for a moment to consider my question, as if no one had ever asked her to confess her honest feelings about this before.

"It feels . . . hard." She looked up at me, clearly wondering whether I was judging her for being a bad mom. "By three thirty, I've already had a big, busy day. I'm exhausted. I've done a thousand things for other people, and sometimes it feels like nobody has done much of anything for me. And then the kids come home, and the evening is all about them. My time doesn't belong to me anymore."

"So how do you want to feel at three o'clock?"

Heather was silent for a few minutes. "Appreciated."

In Heather's mind, the story went something like this: "My life is busy and tiring, and nobody does anything nice for me. The three o'clock indulgence is the one nice, special moment that I get all day long. It's my rebellious, decadent, bad-girl reward. And it's just for me. I need this because I deserve this one special thing."

With that, we discovered a big clue about Heather's food story. She was always feeling tired, unappreciated, and depleted, then craving some type of reward to temporarily suppress those feelings. The problem wasn't with the occasional blended coffee drink; the problem was that the three o'clock sugar and caffeine fix wasn't getting to the root cause of her physical and emotional exhaustion.

"You can have the whipped caramel latte if you really want it," I told her. "Go for it." But I had a caveat, too. I explained to Heather that I wanted her to start looking for other ways to create special moments and feelings of being rewarded throughout her day, not just at three o'clock at the cafe.

She seemed uncomfortable with my suggestion but agreed to try it. She started with small changes, such as swapping that boring cup of plain yogurt at breakfast for a colorful, nutrient-dense smoothie. (See the Choose Your Mood Smoothie Bowls, page 295.) These simple switches sparked a change in Heather that went far beyond a vitamin boost! She felt more eager and excited about food than she had in a long, long time, and that made her open to other changes too, changes that had nothing to do with her food choices. Heather began prioritizing joyful movement and sitting down to actually savor her lunch, even in the midst of her hectic day.

A few weeks later, a tiny miracle happened.

"I didn't get my whipped caramel latte today," she told me during a follow-up session.

"Oh, yeah?" I asked with a half grin. "Was that difficult? How did that feel?"

She shrugged. "It wasn't difficult," she admitted proudly. "In fact, it was no problem at all. I just didn't want it anymore."

A significant shift had taken place inside Heather's mind that created a ripple effect around her behaviors and the choices she was making on a daily basis. Those actions made her feel better and improved her overall quality of life. Her new food story became a practice of saying to herself, "Life is a privilege, and many people appreciate me, including myself. I can create nice experiences and beautiful moments around more than a beverage and not just once a day. I can make choices to take better care of myself to keep me feeling energized and happy."

And just like that, Heather had written a new food story.

But it didn't stop there. Heather continued to make a series of lifestyle upgrades and was starting to feel like a different woman. That heavy feeling of tiredness was lifting, and the stress she had around food dissipated. Even her eyes seemed more sparkly and more alive. She was enjoying cooking and eating, branching out and having fun in the kitchen. As a result, she was experiencing more happiness in just about every aspect of her life.

ASK YOURSELF: HOW DO I WANT TO FEEL?

So . . . how do *you* want to feel?

And not just in relation to food, but in your daily life.

How would you like to feel in your career or business? What about in your relationships and family life? How do you want to feel when you're spending time with your kids? How would you like the environment in your home to feel? What about your body—how do you want to feel in the skin you're in? What feelings do you desire to feel as you go through your day?

Knowing how you want to feel is just the first step. The next is acknowledging what will make you feel that way—whether it's the foods you eat, the beverages you drink, or the activities you engage in.

For example, say you want to feel sexier in your body. Aside from eating sensual meals, you could also take a dance class, wear some racy lingerie under your clothes to surprise your partner (or just because), or take a little extra time to do your hair and makeup.

Or maybe you want to feel calmer in the kitchen. Peruse a few recipe blogs and choose a beautiful dish to make that includes calming nutrients, such as omega-3-rich salmon, fresh berries, and leafy greens, or savor a cup of lavender tea. While you're at it, ask yourself what else you could do to feel calm. Maybe you could take a long, quiet stroll through a nearby park or nature preserve and leave your phone at home or in the car. You could pet your dog or your cat in your lap. You could listen to soothing ambient music or meditate to the sounds of Tibetan singing bowls. You could set some new boundaries with a family member who's been draining you. It's up to you!

Stay open to trying new things and consider some of my suggestions to support the top seven moods we identified in chapter 9. Fill your plate with a rainbow of specific mood-supporting ingredients *and* take your mood boosting to the next level with the following feel-good activities, too. Together, they work harmoniously to help you achieve your desired mood.

Happy

- Blast your favorite best-day-ever feel-good song. Bonus for singing along!

- Watch stand-up comedy on YouTube or Netflix.

- Get some sun. Exposure to sunlight can increase the release of serotonin.

Focused

- Silence your phone to block distractions.

- Play classical music, such as work by Mozart, thought to improve concentration.[1]

- Repeat an affirmation (such as "I am present" or "I am focusing on the task at hand") to quiet the noise in your mind.

Radiant

- Take a brisk walk and get an all-natural glow.

- Roll an ice cube all around your face to invigorate your skin.

- Use one of your top skills: teach, write, coach, mentor, inspire others, do something that makes you feel like you're shining brightly from within.

Strong

- Do a workout or mini workout, such as a few Sun Salutations or ten quick push-ups.

- Perform a generous favor for someone; have a positive influence on someone's day.

- LOL (laugh out loud)! Laughter helps decrease stress hormones while increasing the production of immune cells and infection-fighting antibodies.

Comforted

- Do something nostalgic that evokes positive childhood memories, such as watching a movie you loved as a kid.

- Read a mellow book, one that doesn't have disturbing or violent themes.

- Reach out and connect with someone you love. Text, call, FaceTime, or create a care package filled with tiny gifts and mail it.

Sensual

- Give yourself a mini massage with your favorite lotion.

- Do a deep-conditioning treatment for your hair.

- Take a little extra time as you're getting dressed and choose something that feels especially good on your skin.

Calm

- Light a candle and change into your coziest loungewear.

- Listen to natural sounds like rain, ocean waves, or whale songs.

- Declutter your environment or declutter your schedule—cancel nonessential plans, lighten your load, free up space in your mind. (Instant relief!)

Check In with Yourself Regularly

Make time to ensure you're feeling the way you want to be feeling—and if you're not, start doing something to change that. If you're not conscious of how you're feeling, you'll revert back to some of those less-than-nourishing options, repeating a cycle that you'd worked so hard to break free from. Ask yourself: "How do I want to feel?" and "What can I do to feel this way?"

YOU'RE IN THE DRIVER'S SEAT

Regularly asking yourself, "How do I want to feel?" will inevitably steer you toward better choices—food and otherwise—to create the feelings you want to experience. You'll reclaim your power, take charge, and direct your mood and life experience rather than letting helplessness and overwhelm take over. You're taking responsibility for your own happiness and becoming the author of your life.

Cheat Sheet: How Do I Want to Feel?

Create your own cheat sheet of mood-supporting activities.

Activities that make me feel HAPPY:

Activities that make me feel FOCUSED:

Activities that make me feel RADIANT:

Activities that make me feel STRONG:

Activities that make me feel COMFORTED:

_____

_____

_____

_____

_____

Activities that make me feel SENSUAL:

_____

_____

_____

_____

_____

Activities that make me feel CALM:

_____

_____

_____

_____

_____

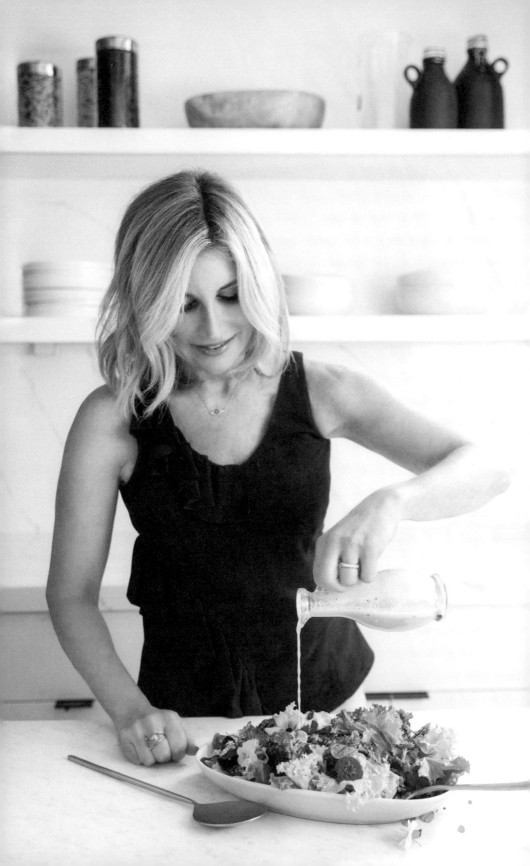

Part 4

WRITE YOUR NEW FOOD STORY

CHAPTER 11

Make Yourself THE Priority

haven't been the priority," Hillary admitted during one of our sessions. A top executive who managed a large team and had seemingly endless responsibilities, Hillary appeared, on the outside, to be the pinnacle of success. She'd broken through the glass ceiling while juggling her duties as a mother of two and a devoted wife. But on the inside, something was missing. Hillary had been putting her career and her role as a mom and partner above her own needs for as long as she could remember. She had forgotten what it was like to put herself first, even once in a while.

"I would love to have more time to do the things I *really* want to do," she told me. "I'd like to actually use that online workout program I recently signed up for and haven't logged back into since. A girls' night out now and again would be nice, too." On the odd occasions that Hillary had made time for herself, she felt guilty. "It's like I should be using that time and energy for something else."

Hillary had succumbed to what so many women are programmed to do: she became a bona fide people pleaser, thinking about the needs of everyone and everything else before her own. She knew deep down that she was fully capable of becoming a better, healthier, and happier version of herself if she made the effort. She also knew that she was the only one who was standing in her way.

Let's face it. Like Hillary, you likely already know what you should be doing to feel better. From drinking more water to getting enough sleep to making time for daily movement, you know what it takes for you to feel good from the inside out. Even though you care deeply about your mental and physical health, those key building blocks are more often than not the first to fall by the wayside.

I understand you're busy with too many responsibilities, and it's much easier to tend to others than yourself. But if your own foundation isn't stable, then you're going to end up collapsing. That's not how the story goes anymore. It's time for a plot twist! It's time to make a commitment, right here and right now, to take that next big step forward toward treating yourself and your body with the same love and care you would give to your child, your partner, or your best friend.

The following food story foundations help make YOU—your mind and your body—THE number one priority. And when you prioritize yourself by tending to your *inner* life, the impact reverberates throughout your *outer* life—positively influencing your family, your relationships, your career, and even your choices with food!

FOOD STORY FOUNDATIONS
No. 1: Flex Your "No" Muscle

Being able to say no is crucial for creating more health and happiness in your life. A lot of women don't realize that saying no is actually saying yes—yes to yourself and yes to the people and activities you really care about. That's a big win in my book, and certainly not what we have been conditioned to do.

Saying no is hard enough when we're being asked to join in an outing or task that we don't really want to do. It's even harder when it sparks excitement or interest. You'd love to meet up with your friend for a night on the town, explore that new business opportunity, or go to a much-anticipated movie premiere, but you know you don't have the capacity to give one more thing your full, whole-hearted attention. And if you can't be all in, is it really worth it? Saying no when you *really* wish you could say yes but know it's not a good idea to preserves your sanity. It prevents you from spreading yourself too thin and not doing anything well, including taking care of yourself! At the same time, saying yes when you don't really have the bandwidth to do what you're being asked can lead to resentment—and that's hardly an emotion you want to be carrying around with you.

Remember, you have a choice. You can say yes or you can say no. Don't make yes your automatic default setting.

Ideas to Help You Flex Your "No" Muscle

- **Listen to your gut:** How many times have you made a decision only to say, "I wish I had paid attention to my gut"? We tend to ignore the soft voice inside or the way our shoulders tense up when we are asked to take on a commitment that we know isn't the right thing to do. Check in with yourself and notice what your body is telling you. Is it saying, "Hell yes"? Then go for it! But don't ignore those initial instincts.

- **Assess your bandwidth:** Before you take on anything new, make an honest assessment about your existing responsibilities and obligations. Do you have the capacity to take on anything else? Would the added responsibility put you on edge?

- **Write down what you would do instead:** Take a minute to imagine your life without the extra commitment. Consider what you would do with the free time that would open up for you if you said no. Perhaps you could do some meal prep or even get to the grocery store. You'll know in your heart if giving up that free time is the right thing to do.

No. 2: Create a Sleep Ritual

Sleep is a superfood. According to the American Psychological Association, getting an extra sixty to ninety minutes of sleep per night can make you happier and healthier.[1] Pretty much everything in your life automatically improves when you're well rested.

Yet the Centers for Disease Control and Prevention say 35 percent of adults still aren't getting enough sleep.[2] Lack of sleep has a cumulative effect that reduces your immunity, slows your metabolism, makes you more prone to stress, raises your cortisol levels, compromises your ability to focus and concentrate, and leaves you feeling grumpy and irritable. Sleep deprivation also kicks into gear the hormone that stimulates your appetite, ghrelin, and blocks the hormone that signals when you're full, lectin, throwing your natural appetite regulation out the window. Ever wonder why you crave sugar and empty carbs when you're tired? It's your exhausted body begging for quick energy.

There's good news: when you do get seven to nine hours of deep, restorative sleep night after night, you drastically improve your overall physical and mental well-being. Not to mention you look (and feel!) like your most vibrant self. The secret to more quality *zzz*'s is a regular nighttime ritual. In just twenty minutes, you can wind down from a hectic day and signal to your body that it is time for bed.

Ideas to Help You Create a Sleep Ritual

- **Plan relaxing activities before bed:** Try the simple yoga pose of putting your legs up the wall to regulate your nervous system and defer to your body's parasympathetic rest-and-digest response. Or draw a warm bubble bath with Epsom salts to melt away the stress of the day.

- **Organize your morning the night before:** Buy yourself a few extra minutes of sleep by preparing school lunches for your kids or your morning smoothie ahead of time. Try overnight oats for a ready-to-eat breakfast treat or gather all of your favorite toast toppings in advance. Same goes for laying out your workout clothes or potential outfit options, as well as packing your bag for work so it's all ready to go.

- **Journal before you fall asleep:** If you tend to have an overactive brain in the evening, spend a few minutes journaling. This simple act of sitting quietly and writing down some final thoughts for the day releases anything that's still stuck in your mind onto the page.

- **Smell some lavender:** Dab lavender essential oil on your pillow or use it in a diffuser. The smell of lavender is scientifically proven to instantly reduce stress and support good sleep.[3]

- **Have a set time for shutting down all electronics:** The light from your TV, phone, and computer triggers your brain to stay awake. Just as you put your kids to bed at a certain hour, put your electronics away for the night at least thirty minutes before bed.

No. 3: Make Movement Your Medicine

There's no arguing: nothing sets the tone for your whole day (and life) better than moving your body in any way that feels good to you—if only for just a few moments. Movement works to heal you from the inside out by shifting stagnant energy and emotions, releasing amazing natural chemicals (hello, endorphins!), grounding you into the present, and energizing your entire being.

Your dedication to daily movement could look like anything from a group fitness class to a long walk to the farmers' market or a hike with your dogs. Movement could also be a few hours spent deep cleaning the house (if that's something you enjoy), raking leaves, or running around playing tag with your kids. Just make sure it brings you joy.

Making time to move each day is an opportunity to connect to your mind and body—and not an obligation or yet another thing on your to-do list. Once you get moving, you'll be glad you did. It is hands down the biggest mood booster, making you feel like a happier and more energetic version of yourself long after the movement is done!

Ideas to Help You Make Movement Your Medicine

- **Schedule movement:** Block off movement time in your busy calendar, just as you would for an important appointment or meeting.

- **See it as a reward:** If you have a really demanding career and are being pulled in multiple directions by your other household responsibilities, designate your daily movement as your protected "me time." By looking at it as a reward for all your hard work, your daily movement will take on a sacred quality that will motivate you to make it happen.

- **Think about your postmovement self:** Help your brain form the neural pathways to develop new and consistent habits by focusing on how you feel after moving your body. When you're sitting in your car after that hot yoga class, actually say out loud, "Hot yoga makes me feel amazing." When you're lathering up in the shower after a long run, tell your body wash, "Running makes me feel invincible." This imprints a memory that will remind you to stay committed to your journey.

No. 4: Drink More Water

Our bodies are 65 percent water, and our brains are 73 percent water, so it's no wonder we feel better when we're fully hydrated. But with our crazy-busy, overactive lives, sometimes sipping enough of that life-giving nectar can easily slip our minds. Even though I *know* to drink enough water throughout the day, I am not always the best at *doing* it. Apparently, I am in very good company, as I ask all my clients about their water intake, and most of them respond with, "It could be better."

But water is LIFE! When you're properly hydrated, your skin shines brighter, your energy skyrockets, your mind stays sharp, your immunity improves, and your cravings dissipate. It really makes that big of a difference. If you're ready to improve your hydration habits but chugging eight glasses of lukewarm tap water every day seems unappealing, there are plenty of simple, effective ways to ensure you're properly hydrated. To receive all the benefits of hydration without having to keep track of how many of those full eight-ounce glasses you've consumed, all you need is a drop of creativity and access to pure, clean water. Soon enough, you'll be on your way to your most vibrant, glowing, and energetic self.

Ideas to Help You Drink More Water

- **Eat your water:** High-water-content foods, such as tomatoes, watermelon, peaches, berries, cucumbers, cherries, peppers, radishes, zucchini, and carrots, will help keep you hydrated and provide your body with essential vitamins and minerals. Juices, smoothies, soups, and even chia seed puddings made from whole-food ingredients are deliciously hydrating. (There are plenty of recipes to choose from in this book—try the Papaya Boats with Lime Chia Pudding on page 231.)

- **Make it flavorful:** Mixing up your own spa water is an easy way to jazz up your regular H2O. Just add berries or watermelon chunks, mint leaves, citrus slices, or whatever combination you can think of. Make it a habit, and you'll never get bored from drinking water again.

- **Bring your own bottle:** The easiest way to ensure you're sipping all day long is to carry a reusable water bottle with you wherever you go.

- **Purify your water:** To maximize the benefits of hydration, drink the purest water you can find. The Environmental Working Group (EWG) Tap Water Database will help you learn about contaminants in your drinking water. As a board member, I know firsthand that EWG has worked tirelessly on this tool for years, collecting data from nearly 50,000 water utilities across all fifty states, cataloging more than 250 contaminants, and pairing the data with EWG's consumer-friendly tips for safer drinking water. All you have to do is go to their website, ewg.org, and type in your zip code to get started. Once you've identified the contaminants in your drinking water, be sure you check out EWG's filter guide to find a filter that is certified to remove those specific contaminants.

No. 5: Spend Time in Nature

When was the last time you stood outside in the rain? Got mud on your bare feet? Watched the dappled light dance through the treetops? Plunged into the ocean or took a walk outside—without your phone? Can you even remember? As members of the indoor generation, many of us spend most of our time—think twenty hours or more each day—inside.

Spending time outside in nature, even just a few minutes a day, instantly clears the chatter from your overthinking mind and invites relaxation and ease into your body. Research shows that being surrounded by trees, grass, and sunshine stimulates the release of neurotransmitters such as dopamine and serotonin to help us cope with anxious thoughts and reduce stress.[4]

If you're thinking you have to go find some remote location to experience the beauty and benefits of nature, you don't! Pockets of greenery exist even in the most urban settings. I live in the middle of Washington, DC, and have found my spots. I go to these peaceful places almost daily as part of my running route or with my pups, and it completely transforms how I feel inside. So find a moment and head outside! Look up. Let the sun hit your face. Get inspired by the beautiful world around you.

Ideas to Help You Spend Time in Nature

- **Commit to a daily walk:** Walking for at least twenty minutes each day is enough to significantly reduce cortisol levels and totals almost two and a half hours a week of soaking in all the benefits of the great outdoors.[5] Fit a walk in as a prebreakfast energizer, midday break, or evening stroll. If you think you don't have time, check in with yourself next time you're scrolling through social media or watching TV and swap in a quick walk instead.

- **Schedule walk-and-talk meetings:** Invite your colleagues to head outside instead of sitting in a conference room. If you're meeting for a call, take your phone for a walk.

- **Do everyday things outside:** Weather permitting, some indoor activities can easily be done in the fresh air. Have lunch on a park bench or coffee on your stoop. Roll out your yoga mat in your backyard, catch up with a friend while walking in the woods, or make an effort to dine al fresco.

- **Plan outdoor activities:** Try glamping, a more glam way to camp, or go hiking, rafting, kayaking, horseback riding, or whatever you love to do. And leave your devices at home!

- **Buy yourself the flowers:** Add a colorful bouquet or low-maintenance houseplant to your home for a microdose of nature. It's not the same as being outdoors, but studies show that even small amounts of nature indoors can reduce stress and instantly lift your mood.[6]

No. 6: Unplug from Technology

You don't need to be plugged in 24/7—you only think you do. There, I said it. In fact, smartphones and other technological devices are designed to keep us addicted to ceaselessly scrolling, checking, and responding. One survey found that, on average, we pick up our phones fifty-eight times per day![7]

Our phones don't just distract us from being present with those around us, especially our loved ones; they keep us from being present with ourselves as well. The more distracted and busy we are, the greater the tendency to avoid taking care of ourselves and prioritizing our well-being. Taking a short break from your phone and turning off notifications from your overflowing inbox or social media feeds are some of the fastest, most practical ways to create a little more space in your life for the things that matter: i.e., YOU.

Use your tech-free time each day as an opportunity to recharge and reconnect with yourself and others, too.

Ideas to Help You Unplug from Technology

- **Leave your phone behind:** Putting some physical space between you and your phone is a foolproof way to create gaps of tech-less time that you can then fill with whatever else you choose. I place my phone facedown in another room during meal times. You can also build smaller gadget-free gaps into your day: consider taking a brisk walk around the block and keeping your phone at your desk, or stowing it in your locker during your workout at the gym, or meeting a friend for coffee (or matcha) phone free!

- **Choose tech-free activities:** It's hard to be on your phone when you're in the middle of a Downward Dog pose or riding bikes with your family. By intentionally scheduling activities into your week that require you to leave your devices behind, you get to be present and enjoy the people you're spending time with and the experience you're having with them.

- **Get off the grid:** Unplug your Wi-Fi for a few hours one day a week or take a weekend getaway to a cabin where cell service is unreliable or nonexistent.

- **Make friends with airplane mode:** Maybe it isn't realistic to totally ditch your phone. Just designate a specific time each day to take a break from the pings and notifications. Start with your next meal and go from there.

No. 7: Play Every Day

Play is an essential nutrient that brings levity into your life, creates space for enjoyment, improves cognitive function, and connects you to your inner child.[8] Having fun is about embracing spontaneity, inviting variety into your day, and taking small moments to celebrate rather than constantly plodding away at a to-do list that never seems to shrink. Remember: not every single thing you do has to feel productive—and playing or goofing off does not make you a slacker!

So many ways exist to add a dose of childlike wonder to your day and leave some of that adult seriousness behind. Of course, there's a time and a place for seriousness. But there's also room in even the most hectic day for some joy and a release of those feel-good endorphins. That's where play comes in.[9]

Ideas to Help You Play Every Day

- **Get your groove on:** To immediately feel less stressed and more carefree, add a little dance party to your lunch or snack time or put some music on in the background while you cook. Go ahead: be your own DJ and turn up your favorite tunes anytime you need a little lift. (See the Happy Ritual on page 213.)

- **Feed your inner child:** When you indulge in the treats that made you feel good as a child, you channel your inner childlike wonder. Slather some nut butter and jam onto your favorite toast and top it with fresh fruit and superfoods for a joyful, grown-up take on the ol' PB and J (page 256), or whip up a batch of Vegan Mac and Cheese with Creamy Butternut Squash Sauce (page 259) and just *try* to keep your inner child from feeling giddy.

- **Be a tourist in your own city:** Imagine you are visiting your town for the very first time and explore some local hotspots. Seeing the place you call home with fresh curiosity will bring about a new sense of excitement and joy.

- **Try something new:** Embrace novelty to pique that irrepressible enthusiasm of youth. Pick up a veggie at the farmers' market that you've never tried and challenge yourself to cook something different. Change your environment by setting up your laptop on your deck, in the backyard, or at your favorite cafe instead of at your desk. Or grab your crayons and enjoy coloring in an adult coloring book. No need to stay inside the lines!

No. 8: Appreciate the Little Things

Cultivating an appreciation practice is the secret to inviting magic into your life. Plus research shows that feeling awestruck is also good for your health and can even help reduce inflammation.[10] By inviting more joy and gratitude into your life, you'll find that not only are you more present with the experience you're having, but you'll enjoy the journey more along the way.

Whenever I focus on the little things, like sipping my matcha latte with the morning sun streaming through the window or watching my son's eyes light up when he walks in the door and sees the pups, my daily existence has more meaning and depth. Appreciation flips the script from what's wrong to what's right. It connects you to your heart and increases optimism. Appreciation also sets the foundation for you to invite abundance into your life, creating more opportunities for those special moments that just make you feel good. Once you cultivate an appreciative mindset, you'll see your everyday life with a fresh set of eyes.

Ideas to Help You Appreciate the Little Things

- **Open your eyes:** Start paying attention to the little details in your day-to-day life: the smell of fresh flowers, the colorful produce, the warm shower, the way your body moves, the feeling of fresh, clean sheets. When you tune into these ordinary moments, you'll start seeing the magic throughout the day.

- **Notice when you light up inside:** Observe how your body responds. Be aware of when your shoulders drop, you crack a smile, you get that warm fuzzy feeling, or anything else that makes you feel alive.

- **Write it down:** Every day, jot down three things that you noticed gave you a moment of bliss. The goal is to try not to repeat anything exactly, so that you force yourself to open your eyes and make the ordinary moments seem extraordinary.

No. 9: Include Your Loved Ones

You may think you have to walk this new journey solo. There may be people in your life who don't support the changes and choices you've been making. They may even seem to be actively trying to sabotage you. (FNA!) Your partner, kids, and colleagues may feel defensive, rejected, or just not know how to respond to your changes. You can show them the way by actively including them in your healthy activities. It's a win-win. You get the benefit of connecting with those closest to you, and they may be inspired to start looking at food and mealtimes with a more nourishing and empowered set of eyes. And, yes, maybe even start rewriting their own food stories.

Of course, trying to involve your loved ones doesn't come without challenges. I've spent the last twenty-plus years trying to get my two sons and husband to support my new food story and hop onto my healthy-lifestyle bandwagon. There have been plenty of complaints about silencing cell phones at the table and too many Brussels sprouts . . . plus lots and lots of "Oh, mom! You're so annoying" complaints accompanied by eye rolls. But the more we went to the farmers' market together, picked out new recipes as a team, and even jostled elbow to elbow for counter space in the kitchen, the more ease and joy we all felt around food. You don't have to go it alone, and a healthy food story tastes and feels better when you're all in it together!

Ideas to Help You Include Your Loved Ones

- **Show, don't tell:** No one likes to be told what to do, and certainly no one wants to be nagged. Instead, lead by example. Simply live your life as a happy, energetic human who knows how to tune into her body and make choices that support the way she wants to feel. Remember, enthusiasm is always contagious—so don't be afraid to spread yours! Show your friends and family how passionate you are about your new food story, and they will naturally be inspired to get passionate about it, too.

- **Make it fun:** Put a new spin on a favorite activity. Next time your sister wants to grab a drink, ask her to meet you for a walk instead. Or invite your BFF over for a flavorful plant-based meal. (The Indian Curry–Loaded Sweet Potatoes on page 209 are a good place to start.) Or take a road trip with your roommate to a local farm for summer berry picking or fall apple harvesting.

- **Be proud of your choices:** Live your new food story with confidence. Remind yourself how much stronger and more vibrant you feel and that you are modeling the behavior you want to pass on and promote. The people we surround ourselves with can influence our behavior in positive and negative ways. We know young children subconsciously absorb beliefs, habits, and behaviors from their caregivers. Don't underestimate the role peer and family influences have on adult behavior. Be the positivity you most want to see in yourself, your partner, your kids, your friends, your colleagues, your community.

No. 10: Live More Consciously

Living consciously means being aware that the choices you make directly impact the planet and that by making more sustainable choices you impact the quality of life of future generations. Moreover, when you begin to think about the environment and the bigger implications of your actions, you move away from the minutiae of everyday life and connect to something larger than yourself. When you zoom out and focus on preserving the big, beautiful world around you, worrying about the extra serving of french fries or the size of your thighs feels a little less important. The bigger picture always provides perspective on what truly matters.

I know you're likely thinking, "I'm not even sure where to start." You're here reading this book, and you're already changing your habits. Becoming a more conscious consumer means you're making the better choices for you *and* the planet. Just like rewriting your food story, greening your life is a process. And just like changing your mindset and eating habits, the first step is to become aware that you want to do better, not to suddenly become perfect. As with any change, one good turn leads to another. And even one small change is better than none at all!

Ideas to Help You Live More Consciously

- **Think twice:** Get into the habit of thinking, "Is there a more environmentally friendly way that I can do this?" A few simple examples include: choosing glass over plastic, then giving your jars a second life; limiting single-use items; walking or biking instead of driving to reduce your carbon footprint; using up all the parts of your produce to cut down on food waste; and bringing your own reusable cup when you buy coffee. Soon, thinking about your impact on the environment will become second nature.

- **Eat more plants:** To limit the disastrous impact on the environment of industrial animal farming, consider swapping out an animal protein or two for plant-based options each week. By giving up just one quarter-pound beef burger, you would save nearly 425 gallons of water. That's enough to fill ten bathtubs![11] And the energy you would save could power your iPhone for six months.[12] You would also reduce greenhouse gas emissions. Skipping that same burger every week for a year saves the emissions equivalent of driving 348 miles in a car.[13] And best of all, eating more plants is good for the earth *and* good for your health, too!

- **Reassess your buying habits:** It's so easy to purchase on autopilot. Instead of rushing to buy an ingredient the minute you run out, see if you already have something in the kitchen that you can use instead. And when you're shopping, stop yourself before tossing an item in the cart just because it looks interesting or is on sale. (Hello, impulse purchases!) By becoming conscious of what you *really need*, suddenly you realize you can get away with having—and buying—a lot less. When you do make purchases, consider supporting brands with sustainable practices. With the push toward more transparency, a quick search on the brands' websites will give you information on their mission and efforts towards sustainability. Then you can choose wisely, with the earth's health in mind.

- **Eat seasonally and locally:** If we're friends in real life or on social media, you know that I am a big proponent of shopping at farmers' markets and supporting local farms.

Ever since I started eating seasonally and mostly locally, I have felt a connection to my food and to the earth that I had never experienced before. And the same can happen for you! Not only do you feel in sync with your surroundings, but by choosing in-season and mostly local foods, you also cut down on the energy needed to transport, refrigerate, and package up the food, helping reduce the environmental costs. And did you know that fruits and vegetables are the most nutritious as soon as they're picked? They start losing their nutritional value with each passing hour. A week after harvest, vegetables lose between 15 and 77 percent of their vitamin C.[14] One more reason eating locally and seasonally is good for you and the planet, too.

Now that you've familiarized yourself with these food story foundations, you can integrate them into your day-to-day life. You don't need to go from zero to sixty right away and then burn out as a result. In order to change your food story and consequently your life, give your SELF (and your health) a starring role. That can only happen when you commit to making yourself THE priority!

CHAPTER 12

Pick Up the Pen

B y this point, you've covered a lot of ground.

You've explored your current food story and how it was formed. You've examined your life to see what kinds of Food Noise are present and acquired some hacks for clearing away these distracting influences.

You've become aware of the extensive benefits of bringing a relaxed mindset and undiluted attention to the table and discovered several quick, simple ways to get the most from every meal.

You've learned about the incredible connection between food and your mood and how you can choose food to help you achieve a desired mood.

You've gone beyond the plate and realized that you can make lifestyle choices that double down on the benefits of all the mood-boosting food and drink.

You've started to think about how to integrate the food story foundations seamlessly into your day, so that you can become your happiest and healthiest self.

You've started to envision a new food story—a new life—that's all about simplicity, ease, nourishment, and joy, with you as THE priority.

You have all the elements ready for a really beautiful story.

And now, the big moment has arrived! It's time to actually write down your new food story—the positive, empowering story that you're excited to step into. The one where you listen to your inner voice and take back your power when it comes to how you think and behave around food. It's your opportunity to rewrite those narratives about "good" food and "bad" food. You can edit the chapter that's titled "You're Not Allowed to Eat That." And, like the late, great writer Nora Ephron, you can choose to be the heroine in your own life.

By writing your new food story, you're solidifying the new way you want to feel around food, your new beliefs, and your new habits. It's your upgraded and improved life summed up in a short piece of writing.

"Do I really need to write it down?" you might wonder. "I already wrote down my old story. Isn't thinking about my new life good enough?"

Just as it was important to write your old story down in order to release it, it's essential to put pen to paper (or cursor to screen) to crystalize your vision and energize you to make it a reality. Studies confirm that when you put your intentions in writing, you're significantly more likely to follow through. The act of writing creates a powerful imprint on your mind; in neuroscience terms, it's called *encoding*. By writing it down, you can increase your likelihood of success. According to one study published in the *British Journal of Health Psychology*, 91 percent of people who wrote down their plan for where and when to exercise each week made it happen.[1] So if you're serious about changing your relationship with food, recognize that you are the author of your story, and you can easily edit it at any time.

YOUR IDEAL DAY

It might seem strange to imagine a lifetime of meals or a future you who doesn't struggle around food. Start by thinking about an ideal day and how that would make you feel. Close your eyes. Envision it. What are you eating? How are you talking to yourself? What makes you feel confident? Proud? Inspired?

For example, maybe you start your morning with some uplifting music and a Happiness Breakfast Bowl (page 203) on the back porch, where the rising sun can shine on your face as you eat. Maybe you make choices based on your intuition and have a sense of freedom because you're not bogged down by a list of "shoulds" and "don'ts."

Maybe you have moments of appreciation throughout the day where you take five minutes to reflect on your victories and praise yourself for how far you've come. Maybe you celebrate a special occasion—chocolate cake and all—without a second spent giving food guilt a starring role. Maybe you go to the hot new restaurant with your girlfriends and talk about what's happening with your jobs, your families, or an exciting event without mentioning the latest detox or juice cleanse. Imagine!

These moments are the backbone of your new food story. Feel them in your body. Get excited by the possibilities! This is a chance to drop every rule, every excuse, and to look ahead toward the clean slate that is your future. We're waving a magic wand here, and everything is possible. Don't hold back. Ask yourself again: "What do I want to do during my ideal day? What are the moments that will help me to feel powerful, vibrant, and alive?" Think long-term. You want to have a long, thriving, healthy life, right? Right!

If you're stuck coming up with specific moments or activities, focus on how you'd like to feel first. For example, you may want to feel strong, powerful, radiant, fierce, loving, happy, joyful, or peaceful. Now, what activities help you to feel this way? (Return to chapter 10 if you need to jog your memory.) You definitely want those to be a part of your ideal day and your new food story, so write those down.

As you write, I recommend using present-tense language. This means writing, "I wake up each day feeling refreshed and whip up a colorful, nutrient-dense breakfast" instead of "One day, hopefully soon, I would like to wake up feeling refreshed and enjoy a nutrient-dense breakfast." Present-tense language makes your new food story feel immediate—as if it's something you're experiencing right now, rather than something you hope to start living later.

Use the following writing prompts to help you generate even more examples of ideal scenarios and activities for your ideal day and to organize your thoughts into a new version of your food story. Don't feel wedded to what you write here, though. As with all of the exercises in this book, this one is simply a starting point. Feel free to add and/or subtract sentences to your story, change the wording so it resonates more strongly for you, ditch it completely, or do whatever you feel called to do. Trust your instincts. It's your story. Do it your way.

MY NEW FOOD STORY

by: _____

I wake up each morning feeling _____.

I start my day on a positive note by doing _____.

I love feeling _____, and to feel that way every day, I _____.

I savor nourishing meals every day.

_____, _____, _____ are a few of my favorite foods—and I love discovering new recipes and ingredients that help boost my mood, too.

I feed my body at regular intervals so that I don't fall into an unhealthy pattern of restriction and binging.

Instead of rushing through meals, I savor my food slowly and invite all my senses to the table. Mealtime feels _____.

I plan my meals on the basis of how I want to feel. Rather than getting distracted by _____, I tune into my body to make the best food and health decisions for me.

I continually ask myself how I want to feel in my life (happy, focused, radiant, strong, comforted, sensual, calm, etc.), and then I choose activities to help me feel that way.

My health and happiness are my utmost priorities. I give my mind and body the love and attention that they deserve.

The food story foundations are part of my daily life. I (check all that apply):

- ☐ flex my "no" muscle
- ☐ follow a sleep ritual
- ☐ make movement my medicine
- ☐ drink more water
- ☐ spend time in nature
- ☐ unplug from technology
- ☐ play every day
- ☐ appreciate the little things
- ☐ include my loved ones
- ☐ live more consciously

When I sit down to a meal, I feel _____.

When I'm grocery shopping and cooking, I feel _____.

While winding down in the evening and getting ready for bed, I feel

_____.

Old habits such as _____ are no longer part of my life. I've forgiven myself for those past situations. They no longer weigh heavily on me. I'm free.

In the past, when it came to food, I believed _____.

But things have shifted. My beliefs are very different now. Today, I

believe _____.

Overall, when it comes to food, I feel _____.

Overall, when it comes to my body, I feel _____.

I acknowledge that my food story is always evolving. The choices

that feel great today might be different next season, next year, or next

decade. I stay tuned into my body, continually asking, "How do I

want to feel right now?" and "What would help me feel that way?" I

make proactive choices to create the mood and life that I want.

I'm proud of myself because _____.

I love myself because _____.

And when I think about the future, I feel _____.

TAKE A MINUTE TO REFLECT
ON YOUR PROGRESS!

You've written a beautiful new food story. You'll quickly notice the
rewards of this big, important work. Your new chapter in life begins
now. In fact, it has already begun. You're living it. And, as the author,
it's up to you to write well and edit as often as you wish.

CHAPTER 13

Let Yourself Be Human

I just don't know what to do. We're celebrating my daughter's high school graduation this weekend at a restaurant that serves the most decadent and amazing layered chocolate truffle cake. I can't stop thinking about it. But I've been doing so well with my new routine. Maybe I should just skip dessert?" my client Lara wondered.

After living a food story controlled by restrictive diet after restrictive diet and nearly nonstop food guilt, Lara was finally feeling comfortable around food and proud of the example she was setting for her kids. She had started listening to her body instead of obsessing over every rule and beating herself up over the tiniest deviation. She'd found a movement practice that she loved and eagerly looked forward to her group Pilates classes. But as her daughter's big day approached, Lara kept returning to the question of dessert.

"Everything on their menu is so fresh and made with wholesome ingredients," she assured me. "It's one of our favorite places to celebrate milestones and happy occasions."

The quality of the layered chocolate truffle cake wasn't what we needed to get to the bottom of, though; it was how this preoccupation with dessert might interfere with her ability to truly enjoy her daughter's special day and spend quality time with her family. This was even more of a priority for Lara now, as her daughter would be leaving for college in just a few months and living on her own.

"It seems to me you have two choices," I suggested. "One: order the cake, eat as much of it as you want, and savor every bite. Two: decide you don't like the way the cake makes you feel, physically or emotionally, and pass on it. But eating it and then beating yourself up about it is not an option, right?"

Lara agreed and told me she'd think more about what she wanted to do. During our next session, she filled me in.

"Dinner was fantastic," she gushed. "The meal was outstanding—including dessert. Yep, I ordered the layered chocolate truffle cake, and it was just as rich and luxurious as I remembered. After a few bites, I'd had enough and moved it to the center of the table to share. And that was that. I didn't give it another thought all evening. It was kind of a miracle."

But it wasn't, not really. Instead of stewing over whether or not to have dessert and being distracted all throughout dinner, Lara prioritized being in the moment with her family and made a commitment to celebrate, not ruminate. She was flexible and open enough to make a decision about dessert that allowed her to stay connected, joyfully and with gratitude. In this case, she gave herself permission to eat the cake, but she could just as easily have decided to pass on it. Either way, no guilt, negative self-talk, or shame spiral. And she learned a life-changing lesson: that cake held no power over her. She was happy to have some, share it, and let it go.

Life is filled with all sorts of challenging moments and unexpected plot twists and turns. They are what keep our lives exciting and interesting! Being open to those moments, seeing them as a natural part of your new food story, and allowing yourself to bend and adapt will make navigating them much, much easier and more satisfying, too. In short, let yourself be human and grant food the power to enhance your life, not control it.

LIFE IS FOR LIVING

Have you ever been faced with a situation like Lara's, where you worried over the food options at an upcoming event? Maybe it was for a work function, a friend's dinner party, or a family holiday. Perhaps you got so stressed out you skipped it altogether—or if you did attend, you found yourself so busy counting carbs and fat grams that you hardly remember anything else about it. You were introduced to the new department head? Aunt Diane is having hip surgery? Who knew?! When you become so rigid and fearful about deviating from your plan that you deny yourself the opportunity to gather and celebrate with other people, you miss out on so much of what gives life meaning, such as cultivating or deepening relationships and making memories. And you might have also noticed that even when you do show up, if your mind is spinning nonstop with anxious thoughts about the buffet table, you're not fully present and immersed in the moment. You're still missing out.

I know, because that was me for a long time. I lost precious time with my family and friends because I was fixated on following my food rules. I can't believe I allowed my rigid, self-imposed restrictions to take precedence over socializing and connecting with people I love. It makes me sad to think back on all of the special moments I missed and conversations I wasn't a part of because I was emotionally absent or stuck in my head.

A major turning point in my food story happened when I realized that I didn't want to miss out on living my life any longer. How about you? My guess is you don't want to, either. Weddings, parties, vacations, holidays, and spontaneous get-togethers nourish us in so many ways. Time with loved ones creates the experiences that make life interesting and worth living. Even if having those experiences means we make less than ideal food choices or have options that aren't on the plan. Life is for living and feeling good!

These moments give us an opportunity to prioritize what matters most to us—connection—and commit to finding a way to stay fully present, without any distracting food-related thoughts. Once you make the commitment to be present, you'd be surprised at how many good ways there are to help yourself stay in the moment, especially if you're flexible. You may choose to have a not-so-healthy dish and enjoy it, like Lara. Or to bring a big salad or tray of roasted veggies to a dinner party so you know there will be options available that make you feel good. Or you may decide to look at a restaurant menu in advance so you can think ahead and get comfortable with the options. Or you could actually choose a restaurant that has something for everyone.

Of course, you may not always be able to plan in advance and be as deliberate as this. Life is spontaneous. Not everything is up to us! There are times you may not be able to eat exactly the way you want to, and that's okay. No cause to drift into that sad scenario where you're lost in your Food Noise. Remind yourself how much you value being a part of the human experience and that being present is more important than what's on your plate. No food shame allowed. Trust that you know how to make your way back to the habits that help you feel your best.

Let yourself be human and engage with the world around you. Allow food to help you connect with others, not to cut you off. In time, you'll find that living life to its fullest is much more meaningful than eating "perfectly."

MESSY MOMENTS ARE INEVITABLE, BECAUSE LIFE HAPPENS

We all have messy moments when we lose motivation, go through difficulties, feel out of sorts, or slip back into old habits. There will be times when, despite the best of intentions, you

- accidentally eat too much and feel uncomfortably stuffed.

- unintentionally eat too little at lunch, and then you're ravenously hungry at 3 p.m. and lose your ability to focus at work.

- eat mindlessly in front of the TV or computer instead of savoring your food at the table.

- hear that old self-critical voice badgering you with Food Noise ("You shouldn't eat that," "You never do anything consistently," "You should be better than this!").

- feel uninspired to cook and order takeout instead.

- are faced with a million other disruptions to your ideal routine.

These moments are simply an inevitable part of your journey. Life is messy. Stuff happens. Of course it does! Plus you're not a robot or a machine. You're not perfect. Nobody is. Perfect is impossible, utterly unattainable. Trying to hold yourself to perfection not only defies the reality of human existence, it keeps you stressed. And we know now that stress is the ultimate anti-nutrient, undoing everything you're hoping to accomplish. Letting yourself be human means letting go of perfection.

I'll admit it. I learned this one the hard way. I am the classic type A personality, control freak, overachiever, and lifelong perfectionist. I spent years holding myself to unrealistic standards that were impossible to achieve, especially around food. Once I woke up to the fact that my perfectionist tendencies were weighing me down and standing in the way of true happiness and satisfaction, I could stop making myself nuts and start living a more realistic food story, complete with messy moments.

It's easy to fall into a restrictive and guilt-inducing black-and-white way of thinking: "I screwed up, so I'll never get healthy!" Instead, acknowledge the progress you've been making to create your new food story and focus on the bigger picture. This will allow you to roll with the punches and get back to what you know feels good, whether it is at the next meal or in the next month. I can't believe that I actually thought one slip-up would make a difference in my life. Ditching perfection and the all-or-nothing mindset is about remembering that messy moments are an inevitable part of your food story.

Messy moments are a chance to get curious and look for the lesson. Instead of being critical, bring curiosity to the issue. Is your body trying to tell you something? Because your body is *always* sending you messages. Tune in and pay attention. Figure out what's going on so that you can be proactive in the future. You may discover that your food story isn't as realistic and sustainable as you originally thought. Is this messy moment because you've set some unrealistic expectations that should be revisited? Putting on your detective hat and becoming curious turns a messy moment into an empowering learning experience.

Messy moments also remind you to keep regularly asking yourself: "How do I want to feel?" and "What do I need right now?" A time-out from your phone and all the stressful news? A nap? A peaceful flow practice on your yoga mat? Give yourself what you need. Nourish yourself physically and emotionally, as best you can. When your cup is full, you'll have the bandwidth to think more clearly and to make choices that will align with how you want to feel. The result? Far fewer messy moments.

This journey is a practice, not a perfect. When life happens and things don't go exactly as planned, learn from it and move on to the next chapter.

What Is This Messy Moment Trying to Tell Me?

The next time you have a messy moment, use these questions to help you look for the lesson in it and find ways to make your new food story even more sustainable going forward.

How long did I sleep last night?
Sleep deprivation can cloud the mind and judgment, making me more vulnerable to a messy moment.

When was the last time I ate?
Low blood sugar can spur the need for a sweet or salty snack to rev up my energy levels.

What's been on my plate recently? Could I be lacking some nutrients?
For example, if a deep calling for chocolate overwhelms me, I might be low on magnesium or energy.

Have I been THE priority lately?
Recommitting to the food story foundations sets me up to make choices that serve me well.

> **Is there a deeper issue here?**
> Maybe I need to laugh or cry with a friend or cuddle up with my partner or dog.

HEALING IS NOT LINEAR

Every good story takes a few twists and turns, offering some unexpected surprises to pique the reader's interest and keep her turning the pages, right? Like a good story, a healing journey is rarely linear. There will be bumps, diversions, and hidden challenges. Every element of your new food story—including these—is an opportunity to grow. Be kind to yourself along the way. You can't bully yourself into better health. Only love brings you there. (Read that sentence again!) Remember: you're only human, and this life is for living, messy moments and all.

Worksheet: How I Let Myself Be Human

I feel _____ about living life to its fullest.

I'm over missing out on human connection because of a "plan." I

feel _____ about being present and connected

at social events and finding ways to keep me in the moment, happy,

engaged, and guilt free.

These are some of the ways I gently start over again after a
messy moment:

_____

_____

_____

_____

_____

If life gets in the way of my meal prep and eating or I decide to sleep in
instead of exercising, I won't beat myself up. Instead, I will:

_____

_____

_____

_____

_____

If I overeat at a meal, I won't let myself feel heavy with guilt or punish myself. Instead, I will:

_____

_____

_____

_____

_____

Whenever I succumb to a craving, I won't let critical thoughts creep in. Instead, I need to:

_____

_____

_____

_____

When I catch myself sliding back into my old story, I won't forget that this is a journey. Instead, I need to:

_____

_____

_____

_____

_____

CHAPTER 14

When Food Isn't the Answer

housands of ice cream memories: Ice cream for getting a good report card. Ice cream for winning a soccer game. Ice cream for not making the volleyball team. Ice cream before heading off to sleepaway camp. And ice cream for dozens of other reasons, to celebrate or "feel better." I can still remember the joy and excitement of piling into the back seat of the car with my siblings when our parents took us out to Baskin-Robbins for scoops of our favorite flavors—vanilla for my brother, mint chip for my sister, and chocolate ribbon for me!

Opening yourself up to all that life has to offer means opening yourself up to emotional eating and the role it can play in your new food story. Whether you ate ice cream or cupcakes to acknowledge a milestone or homemade chicken noodle soup to comfort you when you were sick, you have experienced and subsequently been taught to experience food in an emotional way. Contrary to popular belief, that's not necessarily a bad thing. Most experts suggest that emotional eating is a problem that must be solved in order to have a positive relationship with food. Not always!

FOOD IS EMOTIONAL

When the coronavirus pandemic initially hit in 2020, people were baking sourdough bread like crazy, whipping up batches of decadent cookies, and filling their Dutch ovens with hearty soups and stews. In other words, turning to comfort foods. And there were stories all across social media about how a return to these classic dishes made people feel better in a time of unprecedented stress and uncertainty.

The takeaway: food *is* emotional. You've known this from a young age. It can soothe, evoke memories, create connections, transport us to another time in our lives, and remind us of all the stories that brought us to this one. Every aspect of preparing, cooking, and eating food, from the anticipation of the meal to the physical act of consuming it and the camaraderie of sharing it with others, can spark emotions, such as joy, pleasure, or belonging. We activate all of our senses when we eat: the taste of salty or sweet, the smell of the food's rich aroma, the sound of crunching and munching. With our senses firing, is it any wonder our emotions are engaged, too? Community and nostalgia are deeply embedded in food as well. Preparing certain dishes or coming together around a table for a shared meal are ways we pass down traditions, express love and respect, build bonds, and, of course, celebrate. This is the beauty of food. It nourishes our bodies *and* our souls.

It's no wonder, then, that in the face of boredom, frustration, nervousness, anger, excitement, or happiness, we turn to food. If you have ever eaten for reasons other than physical hunger, you understand emotional eating. We have been conditioned to believe that we need to stop that behavior or, even worse, feel shame about it. It's understandable with the amount of ink spilled telling us to stop reaching for that jar of creamy almond butter, pint of cookies and cream ice cream, or slice of pizza when we're sad. But since food and eating are inextricably linked with emotions, there's really no getting around the fact that they can make us feel things, including better. And that's satisfying and nourishing in ways much deeper than sheer nutrients are.

Let's look at the alternative: emotionless eating. To me, that sounds better suited to a robot than a human being, doesn't it? Emotional eating will always be a part of your food story. What a boring food story it would be if food was just calories and carbs! You shouldn't fight emotional eating. Rather, as you're living your new food story and listening to your inner wisdom, try to understand it and your response to it so that you can include it as part of your story in the most useful and empowering way.

You can eat for all sorts of reasons besides physical hunger: to console, to comfort, to cheer, to dull emotions, to deal with overwhelm, to distract. (I even chose comfort as one of the moods for the "Recipes and Rituals" in this book.) And that's okay, *as long as you feel good afterward.*

Eating emotionally isn't a problem if, after digging into a slice of your grandmother's peach pie or a steaming bowl of your dad's famous chili, you feel soothed, satisfied, and confident. You're connected to your food, savoring each bite, and aware of what you're eating and the way it makes you feel. You're able to appreciate the food for what it is—a coping mechanism—enjoy the positive feelings it brings up for you, and then move on. Eating emotionally with intention and connection is one way to feel good from the inside out. And, to be clear, this applies to eating any type of food, from a tropical fruit salad to a stack of Oaty Pancakes with Banana Coins (page 255) to a decadent slice of cheesecake.

But sometimes food isn't what you're really hungry for, and eating it doesn't make you feel any better. It might even make you feel worse, both mentally and physically. That's when you may want to turn to other coping mechanisms in your food story toolbox.

THE SHAME GAME

Audrey loved teaching yoga. She had a large following of devoted students, but the owner of the studio where she taught repeatedly criticized her about not really "looking like a yogi." Audrey would drive home after class and end up raiding the cupboard, eating whatever was in sight. She didn't even taste her favorite oatmeal cookies, the tortilla chips, and the creamy queso dip she inhaled. Audrey stared down at the bottom of empty packages and jars and then spent the rest of the day beating herself up for numbing out with food—instead of getting upset (actually feeling her feelings) with the critical studio owner and speaking up for herself.

Sometimes when we reach for food in an emotional moment, we're being reactive, acting on autopilot, and searching for the nearest crunchy, crispy, or sweet treat to fill us up and lift our spirits or help us forget. We don't even really want that bag of barbecue chips or plate of fudgy brownies. We just want to feel better than we do *right now*. Problem is, eating in this mode doesn't resolve the underlying issue of your unhappiness, frustration, or other emotion that is making you feel less than. You *still* have to finalize that presentation for tomorrow, you're *still* in that nasty fight with your best friend, your brother is *still* laid up in the hospital, your kid is *still* failing algebra. And it leads to physical discomfort, accompanied by a side of negative self-talk. By now, you know that eating under these circumstances is only going to backfire and create a stress response in your system, which will make matters even worse, not better. (See chapter 7 for a refresher on how stress impacts your system.)

Food is absolutely not the solution if you feel guilty and beat yourself up about turning to it. Or if you judge yourself harshly for polishing off a plate of nachos after you snapped at your kids or spooning up an entire jar of Spiced Edible Chocolate Chip Cookie Dough (page 275) after a downer of a day. Or if you call yourself "weak" and slash at your self-esteem. The guilt and shame you're feeling are sending you a message, loud and clear: food isn't what you need. You're hungry for something else. Time to put down the fork and explore nonfood ways to feed your soul.

REACH FOR WHAT YOU'RE REALLY HUNGRY FOR

Nourishment can come from human connection, pets, music, books, art, movies, crafts, the natural world, physical movement, meditation, mantras, prayer, and an almost infinite list of potential sources. Sometimes, nonfood activities, such as a heart-to-heart conversation with a friend, can lift your spirits or make you feel supported in ways ice cream cannot.

Instead of automatically defaulting to food, take a step back and be honest with yourself about what will really make you feel loved and acknowledged or whatever emotion you're searching for. Maybe it is food, but what else could you do besides open the refrigerator or pantry? What other high-quality coping mechanisms could fill you deeply with connection, compassion, and joy?

A few ideas to get you thinking:

- Call a friend.
- Ask your partner for a hug.
- Go on a walk.
- Take a power nap.
- Listen to mood-boosting music.
- Paint your nails.
- Journal to stay in touch with how you're really feeling.
- Cuddle with your pet.
- Organize a room or clear the clutter off your desk.
- Check back to the food story foundations (chapter 11) and see if one or more can help you feel centered and grounded.
- See chapter 10 for specific actions based on mood.

Flip the Script

When you feel hungry for "something," ask yourself:

- What am I feeling right now? Really feel your feelings, even if doing so is uncomfortable.

- What would I like to feel right now?

- I'm physically hungry. What kind of food would generate the feeling I want?

  Note: It can be tough to fight off cravings when your blood sugar is low. If you haven't eaten enough today or balanced your meals and snacks with heart-healthy fats, clean protein, and complex carbs, grab some nutrient-dense foods that always make you feel energized and happy.

- I'm not physically hungry. What's a high-quality option that doesn't involve food?

TAKE A DEEP BREATH

Will there be times when food is the right choice for you? Sure. But it shouldn't be the only coping mechanism in your feel-better toolbox. It's not healthy or helpful if eating food is the way you automatically cope with sadness, frustration, anxiety, boredom, or grief or if restricting food is the way you feel strong and in control. We benefit most by having multiple options to support our emotional health and well-being. This gives us the power *to choose* rather than to fall into any one behavior by default. After a rough phone call, an argument with your moody teenager, or a scolding from your boss over a lost sale, remember to take a deep breath. What do you really need right now? Food? Or something else?

Deep down, in your heart and in your gut, you know the answer.

Worksheet: Is Food the Answer?

We're going deeper. More questions to consider.

When food does make me feel better, can I give myself permission to let it nourish my body and soul without any guilt?

_____

_____

_____

_____

_____

_____

_____

_____

What celebratory role does food play in my life?

_____

_____

_____

_____

_____

_____

_____

_____

Do I use food to numb out, procrastinate, or avoid uncomfortable emotions?

(If so) What am I trying to avoid?

Do I micromanage or restrict food to create a feeling of control in my life?

(If so) What am I trying to control? And what am I afraid might happen if I stopped controlling things so tightly?

When I'm emotionally hungry for something other than food, I turn to these go-to alternatives:

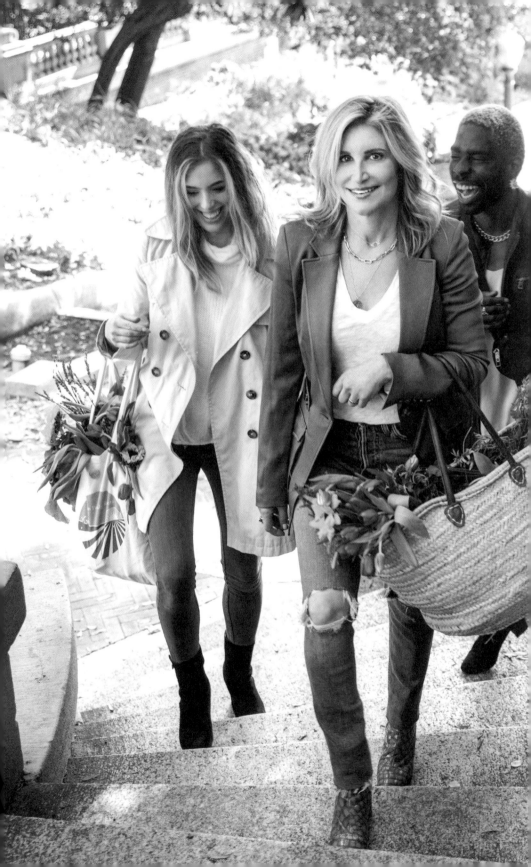

Part 5

LIVE YOUR NEW FOOD STORY

CHAPTER 15

Be Prepared

I magine waking up and having a delicious and wholesome breakfast already prepped in the fridge, ready to go. Imagine taking a midday break from your desk, and your sneakers and headphones are right there in your bag, inviting you to pop outside for a walk. When you make the effort to set up your day, you are telling yourself a new kind of story: "I plan ahead. I make great choices. I am worthy of my own love and attention." That bit of extra energy you spend preparing is the very best kind of self-care: the stress-relieving kind! Seriously. I call it *food prep* and *mood prep*. Together, both serve to subtract stress from your life, so that you can take charge, map out the course of your day, and set yourself up for success.

FOOD PREP: How can you prepare a big, beautiful salad, a vibrant rainbow bowl, or a comforting pot of soup if your fridge and pantry are bare? You can't! That's why making sure you have enough fresh ingredients and mix-and-match basics at the ready is essential. By thinking a little bit ahead, you can have everything you need to pull a tasty, satisfying meal together in no time. Some shopping and chopping are absolute must do's, but I'm all about keeping food prep simple and flexible. Let me say that again: simple and flexible. No hours spent over a stove, no long assembly line of glass food storage containers, no dread of the same dinner night after night. Just nourishing food waiting for future you to enjoy all week long.

MOOD PREP: A stable mood makes it much easier to think clearly and live each day intentionally in a way that feels good to you. The key is to stay one step ahead of stress, the ultimate mood buster. By sprinkling a handful of quick and easy grounding activities throughout your day, you're much less likely to become reactive when something stressful comes your way. These mood-balancing activities can be as simple as five minutes of playtime with your pet, a few deep breaths after lunch, some quiet time with a cup of tea, or whatever brings you back to center. Don't let their modest nature fool you: these mood balancers are powerful and rejuvenating and can keep you in a calm, relaxed, and peaceful state.

When you spend just a little effort planning ahead with food prep and mood prep, you're being proactive instead of reactive. Together, they allow you to run your day so your day doesn't run you, no matter how busy you are.

FOOD PREP

It's six thirty on a Tuesday night. Your meeting ran long, and you've been stuck in traffic for forty-five minutes, getting starving and cranky while you rotate between two terrible radio stations. You stumble through the door, irritated and exhausted. Just when all hope for a decent evening seems lost, you open your refrigerator to find the makings of an easy but satisfying meal that you can have on a plate in less than ten minutes.

(Sounds of angels and trumpets.)

You change into something cozy, and faster than you can get takeout, you're tucking into a big, warming bowl of Cozy Veggie Chili (page 261) with a side of Root Veggie Fries with Beet Ketchup (page 263) and Vegan Cashew Cheesecakes with Purple Fruit (page 249) for dessert. You mentally thank the considerate person who thought ahead and made all this food.

(That person is you.)

It's not an exaggeration to say that making it a top priority to properly stock my pantry, fridge, and freezer has changed my life. It has exponentially reduced my stress, halved family meal gripes, saved time and money, and made it easier for everyone under my roof to eat more healthily. It can do the same for you and your family. When you take charge of stocking your kitchen, prepping ingredients in advance, and keeping your options open, you'll say a permanent goodbye to standing in the middle of the kitchen, fridge empty and cupboards bare, not knowing what the heck to eat.

Stock Your Kitchen

Just as every food story is unique, every fridge and pantry has their own cast of characters, too. I like to vary what I stock in my kitchen, depending on the seasons and what is going on in my life. So before you blindly run out and line all the cupboards and shelves with new items, think about how much cooking you will realistically be doing and how to ease into stocking your kitchen without making it an overwhelming experience. Then create two lists. One is a simple basics list of shelf-stable and freezer/fridge items that you use all the time and just need to restock once you run out. The second is a weekly list of the fresh ingredients that you will be eating and cooking right away.

Your simple basics list might include the following items. Check the Food-Mood Cheat Sheets for other possible staples. And remember to buy items in glass containers or with sustainable packaging as much as possible.

Cooking and Baking Oils
olive oil, avocado oil, sesame oil, coconut oil, MCT oil

Vinegars
apple cider vinegar, rice vinegar, balsamic vinegar, white wine vinegar

Whole Grains and Pseudo-grains
brown rice, oats, quinoa, farro

Nuts and Seeds
almonds, cashews, pistachios, walnuts, pecans, Brazil nuts, hemp seeds, chia seeds,

pumpkin seeds, flaxseeds, sesame seeds

Nut and Seed Butters
almond butter, cashew butter, peanut butter, tahini, sunflower seed butter

Beans and Legumes
dried lentils; BPA-free canned cooked beans: chickpeas, black beans, northern beans, kidney beans

Dried Herbs and Spices
basil, garlic, cumin, turmeric, ginger, sumac, black peppercorns, sea salt, sweet paprika, smoked paprika, oregano, crushed red pepper flakes, Ceylon cinnamon, nutmeg, parsley, nutritional yeast

Condiments
mustard, curry paste, whole garlic

Unrefined Sweeteners
pure maple syrup, coconut sugar, coconut nectar, raw honey, dates

Frozen Vegetables
cauliflower rice, green beans, broccoli, winter squash, shelled edamame, peas, spinach

Frozen Fruit
blueberries, cherries, raspberries, strawberries, pineapples, mangoes, peaches

Sauces
hot sauce, pasta sauce, salsa, tamari, tomato sauce, Worcestershire sauce

Protein Powders
plant-based protein powder, collagen peptides

Plant-Based Milks
almond milk, coconut milk (cartons and cans), cashew milk, oat milk, hemp milk

Flours
whole-wheat flour, gluten-free flour, almond flour, coconut flour, oat flour, brown rice flour, cornstarch, tapioca flour

Other Baking Ingredients
baking soda, nonaluminum baking powder, chocolate chips, vanilla extract, unsweetened coconut flakes, cocoa or cacao powder

Dark Chocolate and Dried Fruit
70 percent (or higher) dark chocolate, golden berries, goji berries, dried cherries

Once you have the basics, then you can focus more specifically on the perishable foods, including fruits, vegetables, fresh herbs, and protein. Write down anything you need that is recipe specific, then have an open mind and purchase what looks freshest and best, which will vary from week to week. Variety is the spice of life, especially when it comes to flooding your body with nutrients and preventing boredom in the kitchen.

In order to make sure you have everything you need, designate a day to shop and check your own inventory before heading to the farmers' market or grocery store. Many of my clients shop on Saturday, then do their chopping and cooking on Sunday to break up the tasks. Do whatever works for you, as long as you have a plan!

Prep Food in Advance

With just a few hours of advance planning and organization, you can save yourself a lot of time, frustration, and meal mishaps during the week.

Some people think doing food prep (or meal prep) means that you're planning exactly what you're going to eat for lunch on Thursday at one o'clock . . . five days in advance. That's way too rigid for me. I have no idea what I'm going to want on Thursday! Do you?

To me, food prep is not about rigidly planning meals in advance or sticking to a strict plan. Food prep just means that I'm prepping meal components ahead of time. I'm prewashing and chopping. I'm roasting. I'm stocking my fridge with great options that I can mix and match in tasty ways. I'm doing all this so that I don't have a sad, uninspiring, and empty kitchen with no options when my stomach is rumbling! Food prep is all about creating more options for myself, not fewer.

Week to week, food prep probably won't look the same. It depends on how much time you have and what you need to prepare in order to feel good about the upcoming days ahead. The season may influence you, too. During summer, I don't cook much in advance, as I'm into lots of fresh, colorful salads and meals. In the cooler months, I tend to have more cooked ingredients waiting and ready to be tossed into warm, cozy bowls. Whatever time of year, always remember: keep it simple and make it fun! Turn on the music, invite family members to join, and remind yourself how happy future you will be.

Here's how to keep food prep simple:

1. FOCUS ON WHAT YOU NEED TO MAKE MEALTIME EASIER. When it comes to mealtimes, to make your life a little simpler and calmer, what would you most like to have prepared? The answer to that question is your food prep priority. Maybe you want to freeze chunks of fruit so it's easier to make smoothies in the morning. Or maybe you want to keep your handbag stocked with homemade trail mix so you don't get too hungry between meetings and carpools. Or maybe you'd like to come home to a big batch of cooked beans and a medley of roasted veggies to add to dinner in a snap. Or perhaps you're happy having sliced peppers, carrots, and cucumbers to easily toss into a salad. Whatever it is, use food prep to give yourself a head start on having components ready to cook and eat.

2. PREP BIG BATCHES OF A FEW KEY INGREDIENTS THAT CAN BE USED IN A VARIETY OF WAYS. Here's a little secret: I usually don't cook with a recipe during the week. Sure, recipes have their time and place. Whipping up a new concoction that requires complex ingredients for a dinner party. Baking Grandma's famous apple pie and honoring her recipe to a *T*. Or adding one or two new dishes to my weekly rotation each week.

But for day-to-day food prep? Collecting new ingredients and precisely following instructions is a complete drag. It's just not happening on top of a full family, heavy workload, and mountain of obligations. For the most part, I use a no-recipe approach to assembling beautiful meals. I keep a few key base foods on hand to mix and match easily amidst the daily madness. What does that look like?

- Roast a big sheet pan of sweet potatoes and assorted vegetables, such as carrots, beets, squash, and Brussels sprouts. Then, throughout the week, you can use these delicious roasted veggies in all kinds of ways. Toss them into a salad. Dip them in hummus. Grab a handful and purée them to make a creamy sauce. Throw a few into a wrap or sandwich. Use them as a topping for a quinoa bowl. With just one sheet pan, now you've got so many interesting meal possibilities.

- Cook up a huge pot of a grain, such as quinoa, brown rice, wild rice, or farro, to add to salads or bowls, use as a base for breakfast porridges, or pull out for a quick side dish.

- Have extra cooked protein on hand to add to lunch and dinner bowls throughout the week: black beans, lentils, salmon, tuna, chicken, veggie burgers, hard-boiled eggs.

Think about the foods around which you center your meals and prepare enough of them to get you through the week. I like this approach because it allows me to prep ingredients efficiently while also keeping things flexible and spontaneous. I can whip meals together on the fly using the different components in my fridge.

Keep in mind, food prep doesn't have to happen on one day of the week. Making an extra serving at dinner one night can ease lunch and dinner the next day—and not in a boring leftover kind of way, either. For example, my family loves to dig into corn on the cob when it's in season. I just throw a few extra on the grill and cut off the kernels when they're done to top a salad or mix up with black beans for a side.

Here's the best part of it all: this kind of attitude has taught me to release my rules, go with the flow, and tune into how I am feeling in the moment. If I can become relaxed and more intuitive about both cooking and eating, then I am certain you can, too!

Keep Your Options Wide Open

There will be days when you forget to bring lunch to work or it's Friday night and you can't even think about cooking. Or don't want to! Rewriting your food story is also about living outside of the confines of your kitchen. Of course, you will go out with friends and family and maintain your social life. But planning ahead for when you're faced with those takeout-versus-cooking moments is an essential part of food prep. Know your options. Which restaurants have selections you are comfortable ordering for takeout or dining in? Check out some menus in advance to get a sense. Food choices are only one consideration. Which restaurants fit your budget? Give back to your community? Uphold your values? Have a plan and a list of go-to places that you feel good about supporting and whose food makes you feel good.

Let me ask you something: When you're stressed out, frustrated, and overwhelmed, how easy is it for you to make healthy choices? If you're anything like me, the answer is: almost impossible! That's where mood prep comes in. Taking a little bit of time to proactively support your mood and stay ahead of stress sets you up for success. Simple, nourishing mood-balancing activities sprinkled over the course of your day keep your mood stable, making it much easier to think clearly and follow through with your good intentions.

Mood prep is a lot like maintaining stable blood sugar. You don't expect even the most balanced breakfast to keep your levels steady throughout the entire day, right? You know you have to eat at regular intervals or else your blood sugar will crash and you'll be irritable and hangry before your next meal. Same here. The positive impact of one activity done in the morning, such as joyful movement or a ten-minute journaling session, isn't going to last all day. By mid-afternoon, you're wilting. But by promising yourself a few grounding practices, you'll help keep those mood crashes at bay and prevent stress from making you reactive when trouble hits the fan. You'll feel better all day long —and, bonus, you'll have extra energy, too. Take time for yourself in moments across your day, and I promise you'll feel more calm and assured from morning to night.

And I do mean moments. Mood-balancing activities are simple but, more importantly, *realistic* things you can do even if you're ridiculously busy. You already know this: that's when you need them the most!

Clear Space in Your Morning

How you spend your morning sets the stage for your entire day. If you immediately grab your phone and start scrolling when you wake up, you're upregulating your nervous system and operating on impulse. You've already triggered your stress response and defaulted to fight-or-flight mode before you've barely even taken a breath! This creates a chain reaction that literally makes you react on defense to whatever comes your way. As you start spiraling out, that all-too-familiar crazy-busy feeling takes over, and you've already lost control of your day before you've even gotten to the office.

If this situation sounds like a typical morning in your home, then it's time to get intentional about how you're spending those first crucial moments of your day. In order to truly rise and shine, you've got to align how you want to feel with the activities you engage in right away in the a.m. We often hear of morning routines, but there's something that can feel a little regimented and forced about that. I've always preferred morning *rituals*, which change the mindset from "I should" to "I will." By ritualizing some of your morning activities, you'll proactively set the tone for the rest of your day.

A morning ritual doesn't have to be complicated or take a lot of time. We live in a world where we're inundated by unrealistic images and ideas of these lavish, hours-long morning routines of "highly productive people" and social media influencers that not only seem unattainable but may even make us feel bad about ourselves. When it comes to food, fitness, and self-care, so many of us have unrealistic expectations.

Sure, it would be amazing if you manage to meditate for twenty minutes, *and* go to spin class, *and* take the dogs for a long walk, *and* savor a nourishing breakfast in a serene environment, *and* blow-dry your hair, *and* write down a gratitude list, all before heading out the door.

And if you are the person who can miraculously accomplish all of those things in a single morning while also working full time and raising kids, then congratulations—because you are a superhero!

But let's be realistic. You have only a few hours in the morning, which makes it nearly impossible to do every single item on your dream wellness list. What's the trick to prioritizing? Choose one to two rituals that most powerfully support you.

For me, that means movement. Moving my body in the morning is the most grounding way to start my day. Whether it's a sweaty flow practice on my yoga mat or a serene stroll through the woods, kicking off my a.m. with exercise helps me quiet my overthinking brain and tune into how I'm really feeling.

Perhaps you thrive on list making and crafting an orderly to-do list keeps you centered and focused, preventing you from spiraling out. Or you may need to sit down to eat breakfast instead of eating on the go in the car, taking the time to feel nourished instead of rushed. Or maybe you carve out a few minutes to meditate just before dawn while your household is still asleep, relishing the quiet to relax your mind.

No matter which rituals you choose to include, a few reliable morning mood-balancing activities will make a major difference in how you'll feel throughout your day. But prioritizing your mental health doesn't stop at 9 a.m.

Spread the Love Beyond the A.M.

Challenges crop up throughout the day: an argument with your boss, a sick kid, a pushed-up deadline, a snarl of traffic. By the time dinner rolls around, the benefits of your morning rituals can feel like a distant memory. This is why it's important to sprinkle mood-balancing moments throughout your day, in the afternoon, evening, whenever!

One of your mood-balancing activities may be to pause for a minute at midmorning to close your eyes, take a few deep cycles of breath, and tune into yourself. Or to eat your lunch outside on a park bench instead of at your desk. One of mine is a little quiet time with a matcha latte. You may also enjoy the ritual of a nightly bath to unwind and prepare for restful sleep, helping you to end your day on a soothing note. Other possible mood-balancing moments include:

- Playing with your kids or pets for five minutes
- Taking a midday walk around the block
- Stretching at your desk or on your yoga mat
- Sipping a cup of tea on the patio
- Pulling out the cutting board and some veggies and chopping away
- Sending a friend a funny meme
- Taking a few deep breaths while looking at the sky

Your mood-balancing activities might be completely different than the ones I've suggested here. (Your "How Do I Want to Feel?" cheat sheet on page 124 may include some possibilities for you, too.) But whatever they may be, you want to keep them as simple and specific as possible to make sure they don't add to your stress level. That way, they'll fit easily into your daily life and help you reduce and stay ahead of stress.

Worksheet: Getting Prepped

FOOD PREP

I commit to stocking my fridge and pantry with the basics and then adding fresh food every [name day of the week]_____.

I will think about my future self and spend a few hours in the kitchen getting ready for the days ahead on [name day of the week]_____.

Some seasonal and fresh ingredients that I want to have on hand this week are:

_____

_____

_____

_____

_____

A few recipes that I have chosen for my weekly rotation are:

_____

_____

_____

_____

_____

When I don't feel like cooking or I'm having one of those crazy weeks, I can find food that makes me feel good at:

_____

_____

_____

_____

MOOD PREP

My morning rituals include these mood-balancing activities:

_____

_____

_____

_____

I will sprinkle these mood-balancing activities throughout my day:

_____

_____

_____

_____

_____

CHAPTER 16

Make Your Kitchen a Sanctuary

Now that your fridge and pantry are stocked, how do you feel when you step into your kitchen? Stressed? Overwhelmed? Just blah? If you aren't instantly inspired, it's time to set a new scene! Instead of walking into a pile of unwashed dishes, trails of cookie crumbs, and a counter filled with gadgets that you don't even use, you can transform your kitchen into an organized and inviting space. A place where Food Noise is silenced, relaxation reigns, and your creativity can run free.

If you're thinking, "Well, I don't love my kitchen" or "It needs work," let me assure you that making your kitchen feel like your sanctuary is not about size, cost, or having luxurious stainless-steel appliances. You don't need to renovate or spend any money. It's about raising the positive energy to transform the vibe and the way you feel inside. You can do that no matter how modest your kitchen is right now. Even if you live in a tiny studio apartment with the smallest, most outdated finishes imaginable, you can still create a magical space for yourself and all the people who eat meals with you, too.

When I moved from my house in the suburbs into the city, I was surprised by how sentimental I became over leaving my beloved kitchen behind. I had a hard time imagining my life without my favorite room in our house. It was the heart and soul of our home—a place for good food, even better conversation, and a whole lot of inspiration. Not only did I raise my family in that kitchen, but it's also where I healed my own relationship with food—and where I birthed the concept of a food story, too!

So as I prepared to say goodbye to my spacious kitchen (and hello to my smaller urban one), I had to part with a lot of the stuff that had accumulated over the years. It got me thinking about the significant role this special room plays in my food story (and all of our food stories). It's the place where we cherish our morning coffee, create new habits, unwind with a glass of wine, make memories, share stories, and feed our mind, body, and soul, again and again. I realized that I needed to set up a new space where I felt comfortable and connected to myself, not distracted and agitated. I had to let go of things that were weighing me down, both physically and mentally.

But you don't have to move to do this. I'm all settled in my new home, and I regularly check in and make sure to notice whether my kitchen stays organized and clutter free. Your personal environment directly affects your mood, stress level, and overall sense of well-being. Outer order can help you feel inner calm.

Use the following checklists to declutter your kitchen, freshen up the energy, and create a welcoming space. When you get rid of dusty cookbooks, rearrange the overflowing drawers, spritz aromatherapy mist, add fresh flowers, and more, the heart of your home will immediately feel bright and inspiring. Once you complete the process, you'll actually *want* to spend more time in your kitchen, and prepping and eating meals will feel like a joyful experience rather than a dreary chore.

REMOVE CLUTTER

Make room in your kitchen for you. Declutter your cooking and eating spaces to change how you think and feel. You don't have to declutter your entire kitchen in one day. If the decluttering process feels really overwhelming, start small. Begin with one drawer. Finish that and then move on when you're ready. After decluttering one small area, you might notice your energy levels rising, and you may feel excited to keep going! Bonus: many of my clients report making better choices all around as a result.

☐ Open your kitchen drawers, cupboards, or wherever you store your knives, whisks, spatulas, and other tools and appliances. Pull everything out. Look at each item. Is it beautiful? Is it useful? Do you really need it? Anything that feels like unnecessary clutter, get it out of your kitchen. Sell it, donate it, or give it away to someone who might love it.

☐ Organize your storage containers. I'll spare you a repeat of the lecture about choosing glass over plastic. Regardless of how you're storing your food, I bet you've got some mismatched tops and bottoms. Maybe a few are cracked or scuffed, or maybe you have so many that everything spills out onto the floor every time you open the door. Cull your collection down to the pieces that nest nicely inside of one another, have matched lids, and still look and smell good. Nothing makes me happier than seeing them filled with fresh veggies and stacked in my fridge!

☐ Open your fridge, freezer, cupboards, all the places where you store food. Pull everything out. Take a look at each item. Is anything super old? Expired? Spoiled? Growing mold? Completely stale? Toss it out.

☐ Clear out ingredients you no longer use. Maybe you bought a twenty-five dollar jar of protein powder before you realized your body doesn't actually like whey. Or you purchased three bags of dried chickpeas because you had big plans for homemade hummus, but you really prefer the farmers' market version. Every time we reach past these unused items, we feel a little twinge of subconscious guilt. Nobody needs that! If it has been six months and you haven't used it, it's unlikely that you will. Toss it to make room for exciting, healthy pantry staples (see page 175) that you'll actually go for more often. Better yet, donate unused food to those in need.

☐ Go through your cookbooks. Do you have any weight-loss cookbooks or diet cookbooks with icky titles, like *Blast Away Belly Fat in Five Days with the Grapefruit Diet*?

Any cookbooks that remind you of an unhappy time in your life? Or any books that represent a stressful or disordered way of eating? You don't need that negativity in your kitchen! Clear these out of your house.

REFRESH THE SPACE

Out with the stale energy and in with the new! A few simple steps can rejuvenate the area and make it way more inviting.

- ☐ Spritz your kitchen with homemade aromatherapy mist— just mix water plus a few drops of your favorite essential oil in a spray bottle. Scents like citrus and peppermint are refreshing and energizing, while lavender and vanilla are grounding and calming. Spritz counters and tables and wipe them down. Spritz the inside of your fridge. Spritz all around. Fresh scent. Fresh start!

- ☐ Sweep or vacuum your kitchen floor. Get rid of dust bunnies. In some ancient Eastern traditions, it's believed that sweeping clears away stuck energy and brings new energy—chi, or life force—into the space.

- ☐ Roll up the blinds. Open the windows around the house. Turn on the ceiling fan. Let as much fresh air and natural light come into your kitchen as possible. No more stuffy, stagnant energy!

- ☐ Carefully sharpen your knives so they're refreshed and ready for action. Buy a small sharpening block to do this yourself, check out a local kitchen supply store for professional knife-sharpening services, or use a mail-in service. Send them dull knives in a secure, protected box, and they'll return sharp ones back to you. Like magic!

CREATE MORE EASE

Don't settle for a mediocre, inconvenient space. Set your kitchen up so it fits the way you use it. No more climbing onto stepping stools or reaching into the backs of drawers for the things you need the most. Rearrange!

- ☐ Consider the top three, four, or five kitchen items that you use most often or that you intend to use often. Are these items in an easily accessible place? If not, move them to create more ease for yourself. If you intend to use your blender regularly, make sure it's not stored up high on a shelf that you can barely even see! Move it down to the counter. I rarely use my toaster right now, so away it went, freeing up counter space.

- ☐ Make sure your key cooking ingredients are accessible. If you use (or are planning to use) lots of anti-inflammatory spices and heart-healthy oils in your meals, move those within close reach. If you store your dried herbs in a drawer, put the ones you cook with most in the front and center.

- ☐ Identify one thing that feels annoying or inconvenient about your kitchen. Maybe there's a rug in the center of the floor that you always trip over. Or maybe the faucet always drips a little bit. Whatever it is—handle it! Get rid of the rug. Call a plumber. Hire someone to help out. Do whatever you need to do to resolve the issue.

ADD LOVE

Adorn your kitchen with things that brighten your day and warm your soul.

- ☐ Put a few treasures around your kitchen that remind you of the people close to your heart. A photo of your family. A copy of Great-Grandma's recipe book. A framed square of cloth from the quilt that your mom stitched when you were a baby. Add items that spark joyful emotions for you. I have a blown-up photo of kale that my son took at the farmers' market when he was in seventh grade. Every time I see it, it makes me feel happy inside.

- [ ] Put something in your kitchen that's just for you. If you love listening to music while you chop veggies for dinner, treat yourself to a nice bluetooth speaker. If fresh flowers make you happy, put a cheerful vase full of them on the counter. You can always find yellow tulips or bold sunflowers in mine!

WHAT ELSE?

Trust your intuition. What are some other upgrades or additions that could make your kitchen feel like a sanctuary? Make your own personal checklist.

- [ ] _____

- [ ] _____

- [ ] _____

Bonus Exercise

Write a love letter to your kitchen to set the tone for a beautiful relationship and proactively spread positive energy so that you feel good every time you step inside. What do you appreciate about this space? How are you most looking forward to spending time here? Describe a few specific moments you can imagine. End your letter by making a pact to create an environment that helps you relax and reenergize as you feed yourself and the people you love.

If you'd rather not write down your gratitude, take a minute to say thank you to this room for continuously nourishing your mind, body, and soul.

CHAPTER 17

Evolve and Stay Curious

My son was on the first all-teen episode of the Food Network's *Chopped*. As I sat in the green room watching him navigate the kitchen while being judged by a distinguished panel of chefs, I felt my heart pounding inside my chest. He was confident and assured as he and the other contestants transformed a basket of mystery ingredients into a three-course meal. Cheering him on from behind the scenes, I was nervous and yet so impressed.

Sure, sharing your passion in front of millions of viewers is no small feat. But I experienced one of my proudest mom moments when Noah looked straight into the camera and answered the question of why he wanted to be on the show: "I want to prove to other teens that cooking with real food isn't that hard." Then he added that not only can cooking from scratch help you feel really good, it is also a great way to relieve stress.

That was in 2012. Since then, both my sons, Noah and Daniel, have gone on to live on their own and are completely independent in the kitchen. They shop at farmers' markets, do meal prep, and prioritize taking care of their health. The best is when they cook for me, which luckily happens quite often. Let me stop and say: I am by no means a perfect mom. Over the years, there was a lot of eye rolling and plenty of frustrated comments, like "Why can't we be normal kids?" But now, they make this mama happy. Happy because, as I think back to that dinner with Steven that almost cost me my marriage, I realize how far I have come.

Back then, I would never have imagined that I could heal my dysfunctional relationship with food and change my entire life. I would never have believed that I could release the debilitating hunt for the perfect diet, learn how to listen to and trust my body, and actually enjoy cooking and eating. All while helping thousands of others do the same and being an example for my family.

I still have good days and not-so-good days. Old eating habits and mindsets that I said goodbye to long ago sometimes resurface. My inner critic occasionally comes out with unkind words and mean criticisms. I catch myself micromanaging my food every now and then. But because I have the food story principles ingrained so deeply into my being, I know that I have the power to flip the script, turn the page, and begin a new chapter. We all have that power, including you!

YOU HAVE EVERYTHING YOU NEED

You have all the tools to embrace and live your new food story. You always did, but now you have the awareness to turn disempowering stories into empowering ones.

Old story: I am so confused and exhausted by everything I hear, read, and have been told. There is so much noise. I don't know what to believe.

New story: I can turn down the Food Noise and tune into the expertise of my mind and body. (That's me!)

Old story: When I sit down to eat, I am consumed with stressful thoughts about food. I worry about what I'm eating, setting off a stress response in my system, which negatively impacts how I metabolize, digest, and enjoy my food.

New story: I invite relaxation to the table and turn on my parasympathetic nervous system with a few grounding deep breaths.

My digestion, metabolism, immunity, and enjoyment work optimally in this state.

Old story: I rush and/or multitask while eating and am disconnected from my food and the people I am eating with.

New story: I give myself and my loved ones the gift of being fully present and connected during mealtimes. I will think of the Chocolate Meditation as a reminder to slow down, savor my food, and notice all the nuances of my meal.

Old story: I am reactive about food and worry about what it will do to me. Will I feel bloated? Tired? Or even gain weight?

New story: Before eating, I check in with myself and ask, "How do I want to feel?" Then, I proactively choose food to support my desired mood. Whether it's happy, focused, radiant, strong, comforted, sensual, or calm, there are ingredients (and recipes) to bring on that feeling!

Old story: I don't know how to make time for myself and my health. I have a million demands (kids, family, work, errands, bills, taxes, etc.) that always take higher priority.

New story: My health needs to be the highest priority, not the lowest item on my list. I integrate the food story foundations as a way of life. They help me thrive, so that I have more energy to show up as my best self and give generously to others as well.

Old story: I can stick with positive habits for a short time, but sooner or later I slide right back into my old patterns. I struggle with consistency.

New story: I recognize that perfection is not attainable. Of course, there will be days when I accidentally eat too much or too little, forget to meditate, skip my workout, lose motivation, or engage in a host of other disruptions to my ideal routine. These messy moments are inevitable and part of the human experience.

Old story: When I feel stressed, I instinctively reach for food to soothe myself. I don't know how to stop.

New story: There is no shame in emotional eating, and it's okay if I use food to soothe and destress as long as it feels good to me. But I also know other coping mechanisms that I can turn to without reaching for food. I have plenty of nonfood options, too.

Old story: I don't want to plan ahead and spend my day doing meal prep. That sounds so rigid and boring. I want to be spontaneous!

New story: Planning ahead allows for more freedom, flexibility, and options, not less. A kitchen stocked with nourishing ingredients that I've prepped in advance—such as roasted veggies, cut-up fruit, cooked grains, salad dressings, dips, and sauces—makes it easy to whip together beautiful meals quickly and seamlessly. I always have future me in mind!

Old story: I lose my cool more often than I would like to admit.

New story: I stay ahead of my stress by building in a few minutes here and there for simple mood-balancing activities throughout the day. Moments to walk around the block, cuddle with my pets, enjoy a quiet cup of tea, or anything else that brings me back to my center.

Old story: I just get so bored in the kitchen and draw a blank when I walk inside. Cooking is so tedious.

New story: I can transform the energy and vibe of my kitchen with a fun decluttering ritual that will change the way I feel every time I step inside. No new appliances necessary!

Old story: Whenever life throws me a curve ball and I deviate from my intended plan (eat too much and feel stuffed, eat processed junk food, skip my workout, slip into a spiral of negative self-talk, etc.), I feel so self-critical. I should be smarter than this!

New story: I can shift from criticism to curiosity and compassion. Instead of judging myself, I can ask, "I wonder why this happened?" I will remind myself over and over that I can't bully myself into better health; only love brings me there.

YOU ARE THE AUTHOR—AND THE HERO

You always hold the pen in your hand—when you face challenges and when you face changes. Because your food story is continuously evolving, characters will enter and exit, new themes will emerge, and plots will inevitably twist. And your story will change as *you* change. That's when you put on your writing hat and craft a new chapter to better fit your current physical, emotional, and spiritual nourishment needs.

The routines that worked for you at age thirty may be outdated when you're reaching forty. The meals that felt satisfying during the coldest months of winter might not feel so great once summer arrives. Allow for transitions with seasons, activity levels, hormones, pregnancy, aging, moves, heartaches, and the rhythms of life. Stay tuned into your body and inner wisdom and trust that you have all the answers.

You are the author *and* the hero of your food story.

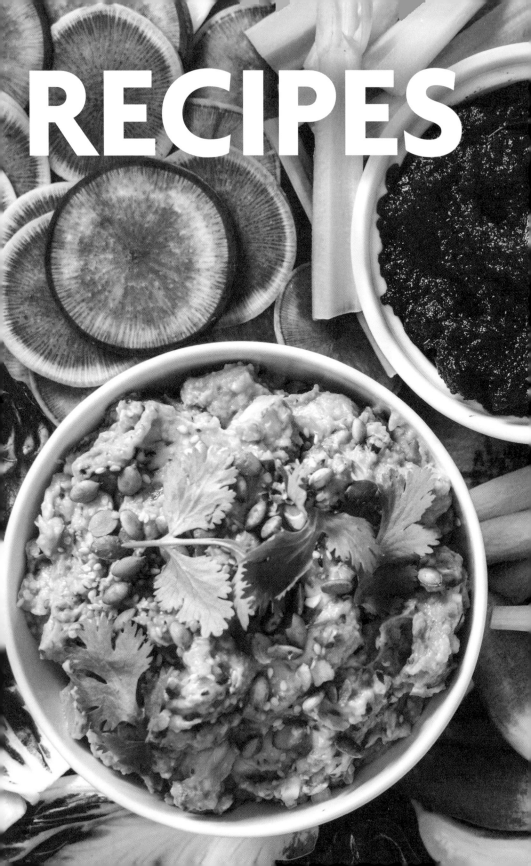

RECIPES

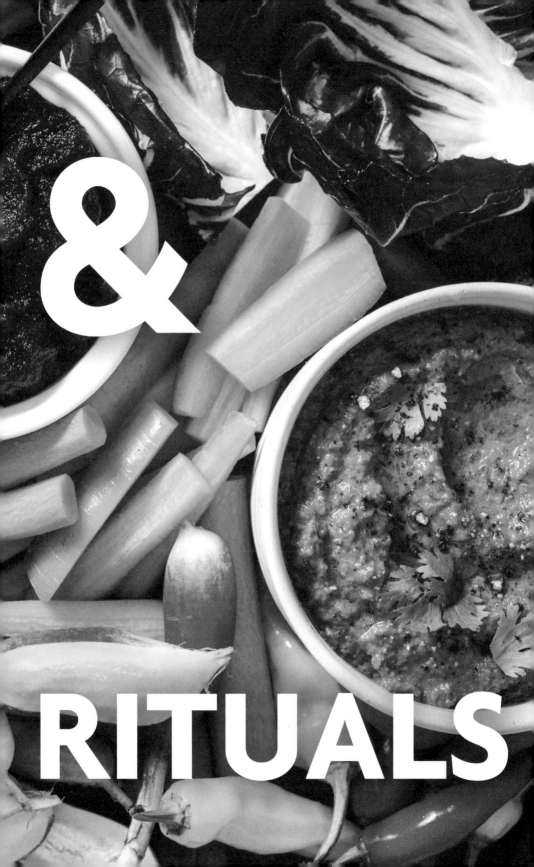

&

RITUALS

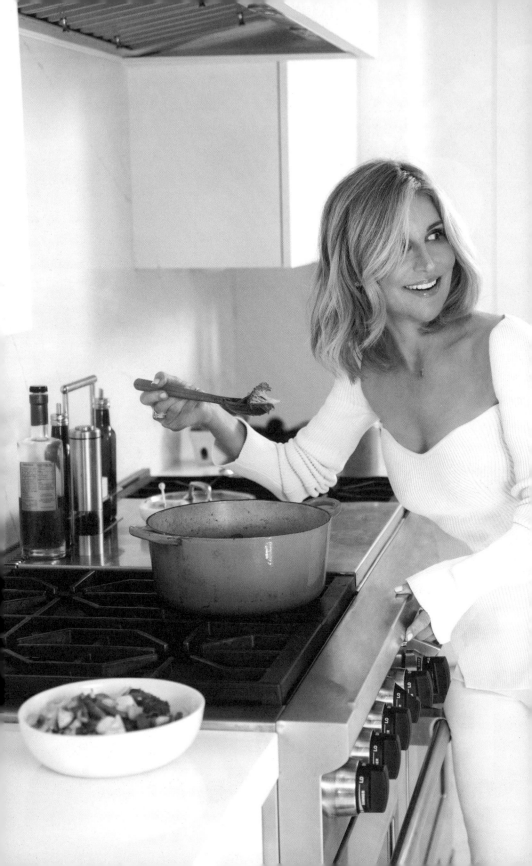

Ready to enjoy food again—enjoy grocery shopping, enjoy cooking, enjoy trying new dishes, enjoy eating? I thought so! With a new food story comes a new approach to food—a fun, science-backed way of eating that puts you back in the driver's seat. No, there is no plan, and I am not going to tell you exactly what to eat (although I do encourage a *lot* of colorful plants!) Instead, I offer you dozens of recipes and rituals organized by mood, so you can easily dig into all the amazing things food can do *for* you instead of worrying about what food will do *to* you.

Where should you begin? Which recipes should you try first? Start by asking yourself my all-time favorite question: "How do I want to feel?"

Whether you want to feel happy, focused, radiant, strong, comforted, sensual, calm, or something else, you can intentionally choose foods (containing specific nutrients) to bring you closer to that desired mood. With happiness breakfast bowls, brain-boosting beverages, rainbow wraps, root veggie fries, hearty and warming soups, beauty salads, and an abundance of chocolate, it may be hard for you to choose!

At first, eating this way might seem like learning a new language. You might think, "I want to feel focused. So wait . . . huh . . . um,

I forget. What am I supposed to eat? Tomatoes? Or walnuts? Some other food? I don't remember!" But pretty quickly, you'll get the hang of things. You'll start tossing cacao nibs and leafy greens into your morning smoothie when you need a happiness boost or add in mango and spinach when you want to feel radiant.

Once upon a time, you had no idea what a carbohydrate, protein, or fat was, but eventually you caught on. The same thing will happen with the food-mood connection. I promise you, it gets easier, and soon you'll know exactly which foods to choose for what desired outcome. This is not something to feel obsessive or stressed about. Totally the opposite. You're here to experience less stress—and more ease and joy—when it comes to food. So have fun with it!

Remember: you are unique, and nobody can tell you what's right for you but you. Tune into your body and let your inner wisdom guide you to the recipes and ingredients that speak to you. Try a new spice, an unfamiliar ingredient, or a different flavor combination. An open mind and an adventurous spirit will lead you to an exciting new chapter! Food Noise, outdated beliefs, and disempowering stories no longer have a place at your table. Instead, invite in relaxation, connection, and your trustworthy intuition.

So how do you want to feel? Turn the pages for a recipe, a ritual, or both to generate the feeling you want.

Let's cook and eat!

HAPPY

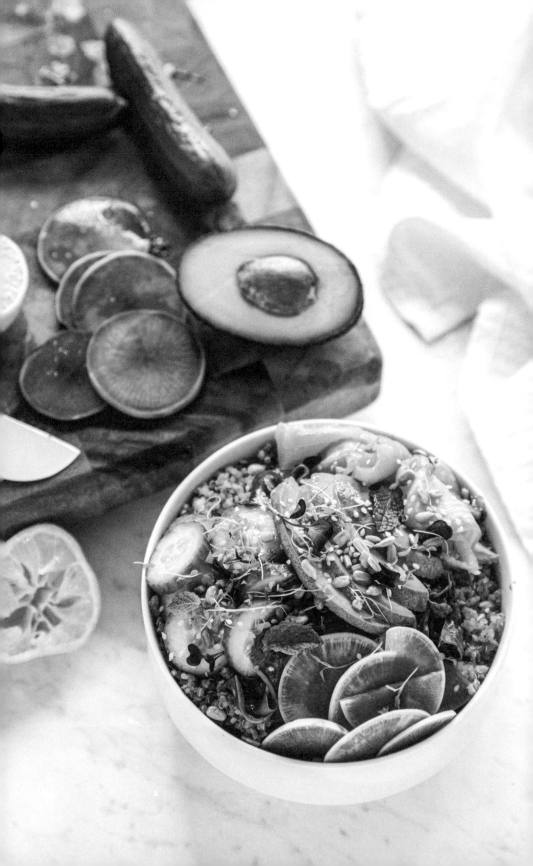

Happiness Breakfast Bowls

The inspiration for this recipe comes from my son Noah, who knows how to start the day out on the right note! Quinoa increases the production of the happiness hormone serotonin, and the garlicky leafy greens are a rich source of magnesium, also known as the anti-stress mineral. Creamy avocado and toasted seeds add depression-fighting omega-3s, while the turmeric contains compounds to uplift your mood. For an extra hit of protein—which is key for balancing blood sugar—top off this dish with 1 or 2 soft-boiled eggs, ¼ cup sliced smoked salmon, or ¼ cup cooked beans.

Tip: Make the tahini dressing and quinoa mixture in advance, so all you have to do is sauté the greens and load up your bowl the next morning.

BREAKFAST BOWLS

⅔ cup uncooked quinoa

1 tsp ground turmeric

fine sea salt and freshly ground black pepper

2 Tbsp finely chopped fresh mint leaves

2 Tbsp finely chopped fresh cilantro leaves

2 green onions, thinly sliced

1 Tbsp extra-virgin olive oil

1 large clove garlic, minced (optional)

6 to 8 oz chopped fresh greens, such as kale, Swiss chard, or collard greens

½ cup very thinly sliced English or Persian cucumber

¼ cup very thinly sliced radishes

1 avocado, pitted, peeled, and thinly sliced

¼ cup toasted seeds, such as pumpkin seeds, hemp seeds, and/or sesame seeds

1 Tbsp microgreens, for garnish (optional)

TAHINI DRESSING

¼ cup tahini

¼ cup fresh lemon juice

2 Tbsp extra-virgin olive oil

¼ tsp fine sea salt

1. To make the tahini dressing, in a small bowl, whisk together the tahini, lemon juice, olive oil, and salt. Thin with 2 tablespoons of water, or enough to create a pourable consistency. Set aside.

2. In a saucepan, combine the quinoa with 1⅓ cups water, the turmeric, and ½ teaspoon salt. Bring to a boil over high heat, stirring once or twice. Reduce the heat to low, cover, and simmer until the quinoa is tender and the water has been completely absorbed, about 15 minutes. Wait 5 minutes, then remove the lid and fluff with a fork. Transfer to a bowl and toss with 2 tablespoons of the tahini dressing until the grains are evenly coated. Add 1 tablespoon each of the mint and cilantro and half of the green onions. Set aside.

Happiness Breakfast Bowls (cont.)

3. In a clean saucepan over medium heat, warm the oil and garlic until the garlic starts to sizzle. Add the greens, season with salt and pepper, and cook, stirring, until the greens are wilted and tender, 2 to 5 minutes, depending on the type of greens you are using. Reduce the heat to low if the greens are cooking too quickly. Divide the greens between 4 shallow bowls.

4. Top the greens with the quinoa mixture, dividing it evenly among the bowls. Next add the cucumber, radish, avocado, and seeds, then drizzle with some of the tahini dressing. Garnish with the remaining mint and cilantro and microgreens, if using. Serve immediately.

Choose Your Own Adventure Granola

The smell of freshly baked granola is enough to put you in a good mood! High in fiber to keep your gut happy and energy level steady, oats are also loaded with mood-enhancing selenium. Toss in nuts and seeds for an added dose of relaxing magnesium and uplifting omega-3s. Use this recipe as a base, then personalize it by mixing and matching different combinations of dried fruit with nuts and seeds.

Tip: Some of my favorite combinations of nuts and dried fruit include blueberries and walnuts, cranberries and pecans, cherries and almonds, mangoes and Brazil nuts, or apples and almonds.

INGREDIENTS

2 cups old-fashioned rolled oats

⅓ cup uncooked quinoa

½ cup chopped nuts (almonds, pecans, walnuts, or Brazil nuts)

¼ cup pumpkin seeds

2 Tbsp chia seeds or flaxseeds

⅓ cup unsweetened coconut flakes

¼ cup unsalted, unsweetened almond butter

¼ cup melted coconut oil

¼ cup chopped, pitted dates

3 Tbsp maple syrup

½ tsp ground cinnamon

1 tsp vanilla extract

½ tsp fine sea salt

½ cup dried fruit (optional)

your favorite dairy or non-dairy yogurt, for serving

mixed berries, for serving

1. Preheat the oven to 300°F. Line a large rimmed baking sheet with parchment paper.

2. In a large bowl, toss together the oats, quinoa, nuts, seeds, and coconut flakes. In the bowl of a food processor, process together the almond butter, coconut oil, dates, maple syrup, cinnamon, vanilla, and salt until well combined, about 1 minute. (Alternatively, chop the dates very fine and stir together the ingredients in a bowl.)

3. Pour the almond butter mixture over the oat mixture and mix until well combined and the oat mixture is coated evenly. Spread and press the mixture into an even layer on the prepared baking sheet. Bake, stirring once or twice, until the granola smells toasty and looks golden brown, about 20 to 25 minutes.

4. Transfer the baking sheet to a wire rack to cool the granola completely, stirring once or twice while it is cooling. (The granola will be slightly wet when hot, but then will cool and become crisp.) Add the dried fruit, if using. Serve with dairy or non-dairy yogurt and fresh berries, enjoy with a plant-based milk and fresh fruit, or just eat by the handful!

Bean Tostadas with Shredded Kale–Cabbage Slaw and Avocado

MAKES 4 TO 6 SERVINGS

Using dried beans in these next-level tostadas really makes a difference, especially if you can get your hands on special heirloom varieties. In addition to being high in fiber and plant-based protein, beans are a good source of mood-lifting nutrients, including B vitamins, zinc, and magnesium. The symphony of flavors comes together when combined with the shredded kale–cabbage slaw and avocado, also happiness-boosting superstars.

Tip: Soak the dried beans overnight to speed up the cooking time. You can also quick-soak the beans in boiling water for 30 minutes before cooking.

SHREDDED KALE–CABBAGE SLAW AND AVOCADO

3 cups finely shredded red and/or green cabbage

1 cup finely shredded kale leaves

1 medium carrot, peeled and finely shredded

½ jalapeño, seeded (if desired) and minced

¼ cup finely chopped fresh cilantro, plus sprigs for garnish

1 Tbsp avocado oil

1 lime

1 avocado, pitted, peeled, and thinly sliced

BEANS

1 Tbsp avocado oil

⅓ cup finely chopped yellow onion (about ¼ onion)

2 cloves garlic, smashed

1 cup (about 7 oz) dried pinto beans or heirloom beans, such as yellow eye or Mayocoba, soaked overnight in cold water

4 cups reduced-sodium vegetable broth or water

½ tsp ground cumin

fine sea salt and freshly ground pepper

4 to 6 corn tostadas (each 5 to 6 inches in diameter), for serving

1. In a saucepan over medium-low heat, warm 1 tablespoon of avocado oil. Add the onion and garlic and cook, stirring occasionally, until the onion softens, about 5 minutes. Drain the beans and add them to the pot, stirring to combine. Add the broth or water and cumin. Increase the heat to high and bring to a boil. Reduce the heat to medium-low and simmer, stirring occasionally, for 30 minutes. Reduce the heat to low and stir in ½ teaspoon salt. Partially cover the pan and continue to cook, stirring occasionally, until the beans are slightly saucy and very tender but not mushy, 30 to 60 minutes longer. (The amount of time will depend on the age and size of the beans.) If the beans start to dry out, add a little boiling water; if the beans are too saucy, remove the pan lid and turn the heat up slightly. They will thicken as they cool.

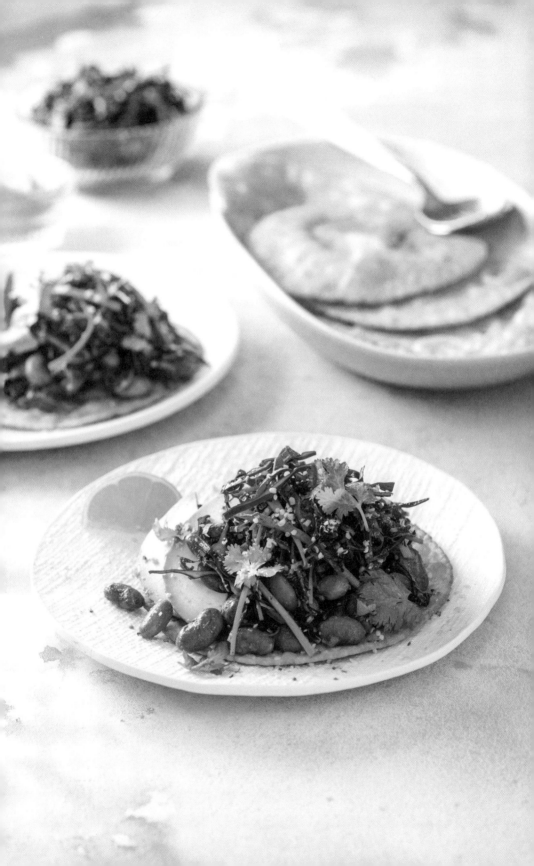

Bean Toastadas (cont.)

2. To make the slaw, toss together the cabbage, kale, carrot, jalapeño, and chopped fresh cilantro in a medium bowl. Drizzle with 1 tablespoon avocado oil and the juice of ½ the lime. Season with salt and pepper and toss again. (The slaw can be made up to 2 hours in advance and stored in an airtight container in the refrigerator.)

3. Cut the remaining ½ lime into 4 wedges. Toast the corn tostadas in the oven, if desired, and rewarm the beans over low heat. Place a tostada on each individual plate. Using a slotted spoon, divide the beans among the tostadas. Top each serving with a tangle of the slaw, garnish with sliced avocado and a sprig of cilantro, add a wedge of lime to each, and serve.

Indian Curry-Loaded Sweet Potatoes

MAKES 4 SERVINGS

Spiced Indian-style chickpea and spinach curry tops roasted sweet potatoes in this hearty plant-based meal. The bright colors and bold flavors make you feel good just looking at it! Sweet potatoes are packed with mood-boosting nutrients, including beta carotene and vitamin C, and can help produce serotonin, known as the happy chemical. Coconut milk adds decadent creaminess to the curry, and a splash of lemon juice brightens it all up. This is like two recipes in one: you can serve the curry on its own or over steamed brown rice or quinoa, or simply use the directions for baking the sweet potatoes and serve with any colorful topping you like.

INGREDIENTS

4 sweet potatoes (each about 8 oz)

1 Tbsp coconut oil, avocado oil, or extra-virgin olive oil

½ yellow onion, finely chopped

2 cloves garlic, minced

1 tsp peeled and grated fresh ginger

1 tsp crushed red pepper flakes, or to taste

1 tsp ground cumin

½ tsp ground coriander

½ tsp ground turmeric

½ tsp fine sea salt

1 15.5-oz can or jar chickpeas, rinsed and drained (about 1½ cups)

juice of ½ lemon

1 13.5-oz can coconut milk

2 oz baby spinach

¼ cup packed chopped fresh cilantro

1. To bake the sweet potatoes, preheat the oven to 350°F. Scrub the potatoes and poke each one all over with a paring knife. Place on a parchment-lined baking sheet. Bake until very soft when pressed, about 50 minutes. (Timing may vary, depending on the freshness of the vegetable.)

2. Meanwhile, make the curry: In a medium saucepan over medium heat, warm the oil. Cook the onion, stirring occasionally, until softened, about 4 minutes. Add the garlic, ginger, and pepper flakes and cook until fragrant, about 1 minute. Reduce the heat to low and stir in the cumin, coriander, turmeric, and salt. Add the chickpeas and lemon juice and stir to combine, then stir in the coconut milk. Increase the heat to medium-high and bring to a gentle boil, then reduce the heat to medium-low and simmer, stirring occasionally, until the mixture is fragrant, about 15 minutes. Stir in the spinach and half of the cilantro. Simmer, stirring, until the spinach is wilted and warmed through. Remove from the heat and cover to keep warm.

3. When the sweet potatoes are ready, divide them between individual plates. Split each sweet potato lengthwise down the middle and press the ends to open it up. Ladle the curry into the sweet potatoes, dividing it evenly (about ¾ cup each). Garnish with the remaining cilantro and serve.

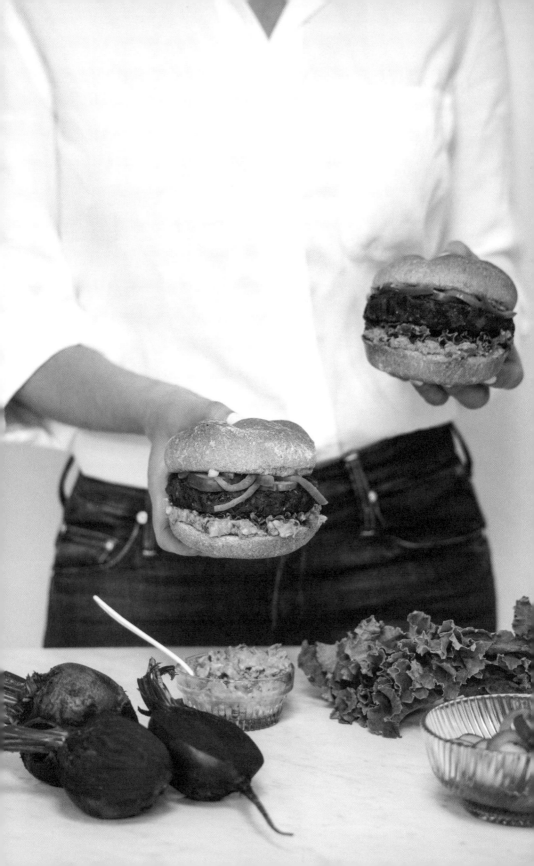

Can't Be Beet Burgers with Quick Pickled Onions and Chipotle-Avocado Spread

MAKES 6 BURGERS

A truly revelatory flavor combination? Smoke-kissed vegan burger, vinegary pickled vegetables, and spicy chipotle-avocado spread! The patties are a magical mixture of raw shredded beets, mashed black beans, and quinoa spiced with smoked paprika and cumin. Beets are energizing from the inside out! They are an excellent source of betaine, a nutrient found to help lower depressive symptoms, and their vibrant color is revitalizing, too. Even if you're not a beet fan, be open-minded and try this!

Tip: The uncooked burgers can be frozen in an airtight container, separated by parchment paper, for up to 1 month. Let thaw at room temperature for 30 minutes before cooking and add a few minutes' cooking time. They make a quick and easy midweek meal.

QUICK PICKLED ONIONS

½ small red onion, thinly sliced

2 cups boiling water

¼ cup unseasoned rice vinegar

1 tsp coconut sugar

¼ tsp dried oregano

¼ tsp ground cumin

⅛ tsp fine sea salt

3-inch piece English cucumber, cut into ¼-inch-thick slices

CHIPOTLE-AVOCADO SPREAD

1 tsp minced chipotle in adobo sauce, plus 1 tsp adobo sauce

1 ripe avocado, pitted, peeled, and chopped

1 tsp lime juice

fine sea salt

BEET BURGERS

1 15.5-oz can black beans, rinsed and drained (about 1½ cups cooked beans)

1 cup finely grated beets

½ cup cooked quinoa

2 Tbsp finely grated yellow onion

2 Tbsp oat flour

1 Tbsp Dijon mustard

½ tsp smoked paprika

½ tsp cumin

½ tsp fine sea salt

¼ tsp freshly ground pepper

1 Tbsp avocado oil, olive oil, or coconut oil

6 whole-wheat or gluten-free burger buns, toasted, or 6 crisp lettuce leaves

Can't Be Beet Burgers (cont.)

1. To make the pickles, put the red onion slices in a small saucepan and pour the boiling water over them. Let sit for 5 minutes, then drain and rinse well. Combine the vinegar, sugar, oregano, cumin, and salt in the saucepan and bring to a boil over medium-high heat. Add the blanched onion slices and cucumber, stir to combine, and remove from the heat. Transfer to an airtight container and set aside to cool to room temperature, stirring every so often. Cover and refrigerate for at least 30 minutes or up to 3 days before using.

2. To make the burger patties, put the black beans in a medium bowl. Using a fork, mash the beans into a thick, coarse purée. Measure out the shredded beet, then wrap in paper towels and squeeze out as much liquid as you can. Add to the beans. Add the remaining ingredients except the oil and stir until evenly combined. Divide the mixture into 6 equal portions and press each portion into a patty. Set aside.

3. To make the spread, in a small bowl, mash the chipotle and adobo sauce, avocado, lime juice, and salt together until smooth and well combined.

4. To cook the burgers, heat a large, well-seasoned skillet over medium-low heat. Add the oil, swirl to coat the pan, then add the patties in a single layer. (You may need to do this in batches.) Cook the patties, carefully turning once or twice, until nicely browned and crisp on both sides and heated through, about 8 minutes.

5. To assemble, smear the cut sides of each bun with the spread. Layer the bottom bun with a patty, some of the pickles, a lettuce leaf, and the top bun. Serve warm. (If using a lettuce leaf in place of a bun, layer the spread, beet burger, and pickles inside the lettuce leaf before wrapping it around.)

HAPPY FOOD-MOOD CHEAT SHEET

Quick tip: Choose colorful plants, healthy fats, and complex carbs to uplift your mood.

avocado	fatty fish
beans	fermented foods
beets	hemp seeds
berries	leafy greens
cacao	matcha tea
chia seeds	sweet potatoes
dark chocolate	whole grains

HAPPY RITUAL

Dance Break!

Time to get moving! Need some motivation? Here it is: When we move around in any way, we're more patient, more focused, and more relaxed. Movement releases endorphins, which can reduce stress, bust bad moods, and promote restful sleep. So turn on your favorite tunes (music is another mood booster!) and have a one-person dance party in your kitchen or invite your family members to join.

Feel like you've got zero dance skills and you look like a total goofball? Ha! I can relate. But remember, you don't need to look like a professional Broadway performer—the whole point is just to move around and feel good. Do it for one song, even if it feels strange or uncomfortable. You'll instantly notice your spirits lift. Singing into your spatula is optional!

FOCUSED

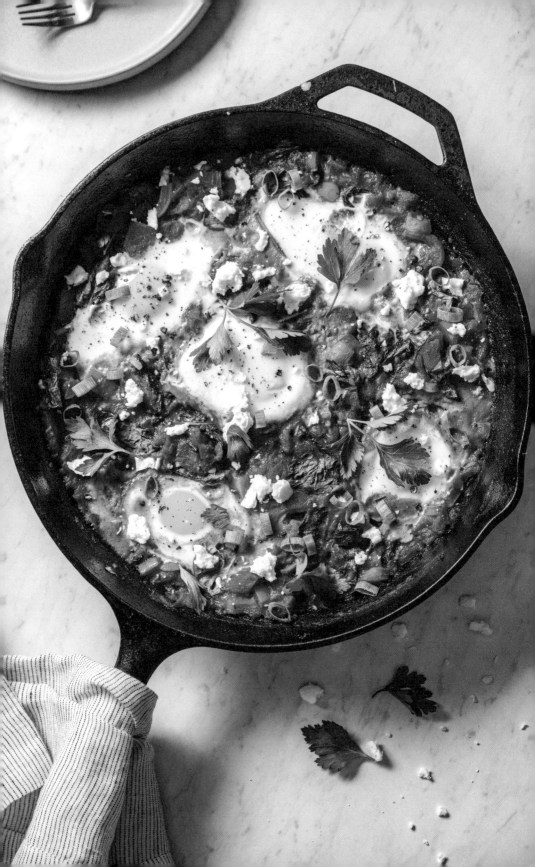

Skillet Shakshuka

Shakshuka is a fragrant pepper- and tomato-based Middle Eastern egg dish. The eggs are baked into the warm sauce, then topped with fresh herbs, green onions, and crumbled feta cheese. Choline, a key nutrient found in egg yolks, helps support concentration and mental focus. The garlic and anti-inflammatory spices enliven the sauce and can help reduce signs of cognitive decline. You can make the sauce up to two days in advance—just warm it back up before you add the eggs.

Tip: For a vegan version, omit the eggs, add seared cubes of tofu, and use vegan cheese.

INGREDIENTS

2 Tbsp extra-virgin olive oil

¼ small yellow onion, finely chopped

1 red or orange bell pepper, cored, seeded, and chopped

2 cloves garlic, minced

1 tsp sweet paprika

½ tsp chopped fresh or dried oregano

¼ tsp ground cumin

fine sea salt and freshly ground black pepper

2 cups canned whole tomatoes, with juices

1 cup baby spinach

4 to 6 large eggs

¼ cup crumbled feta or vegan cheese

1 thinly sliced green onion, both white and green parts

3 Tbsp chopped fresh cilantro or flat-leaf Italian parsley

1. Preheat the oven to 400°F. In a 10-inch ovenproof skillet over medium heat, warm the oil. Add the onion and bell pepper and cook, stirring occasionally, until the vegetables are tender and starting to brown, about 7 minutes.

2. Stir in the garlic, paprika, oregano, cumin, ½ teaspoon salt, and a few grinds of pepper. Cook just until fragrant, about 30 seconds. Reduce the heat to medium-low and add the canned tomatoes with their juices, breaking them up with your hands as you add them. Stir to combine.

3. Bring the mixture to a simmer, then stir in the spinach. Continue to simmer until the spinach is wilted and the sauce is fragrant, about 5 minutes. (If the sauce is too thick, add a few tablespoons of water.)

4. Use the back of a big spoon to create 4 to 6 wells in the tomato mixture. Crack an egg into each well and season with a little salt and pepper. Transfer the pan to the oven and bake until the egg whites are barely cooked and the yolks are still runny, about 12 minutes. (The eggs will continue to cook while you are garnishing.)

5. Sprinkle with the feta cheese, green onions, and cilantro or Italian parsley. Serve immediately.

Glazed Salmon with Ginger, Lemon, and Tamari

MAKES 4 SERVINGS

This flavorful dish is so quick and easy, it's certain to become a weeknight staple. Packed with omega-3 fatty acids to support memory, salmon also contains vitamin B-12, which can help produce brain chemicals that enhance your overall mood. For even more brain-boosting benefits, serve the salmon and zesty sauce over steamed quinoa with sautéed leafy greens. Any leftover salmon is great atop a salad the next day.

Tip: Be sure to use reduced-sodium tamari or soy, or the sauce will be overly salty. You can leave out the maple syrup, but it helps balance the brightness of the other ingredients.

INGREDIENTS

4 salmon fillets (1½ pounds), pin bones removed

½ cup reduced-sodium tamari or soy sauce

finely grated zest of 1 lemon

¼ cup fresh lemon juice

1 Tbsp maple syrup

2 tsp finely grated fresh ginger

1. Place the salmon skin-side up in a baking dish just large enough to hold it in a single layer. In a bowl, whisk together the tamari, lemon zest and juice, maple syrup, and ginger. Pour over the salmon, turning to coat it in the marinade, and return it to skin-side up. Set aside to marinate at room temperature for 10 minutes.

2. Preheat the oven to 420°F. Turn the salmon skin-side down. Bake the salmon until just barely opaque throughout, 10 to 12 minutes (depending on the thickness of the fillet and how you like it cooked).

3. Transfer the salmon to a serving plate, discarding the skin. Transfer the sauce to a small bowl or pitcher. Serve the salmon with the sauce alongside.

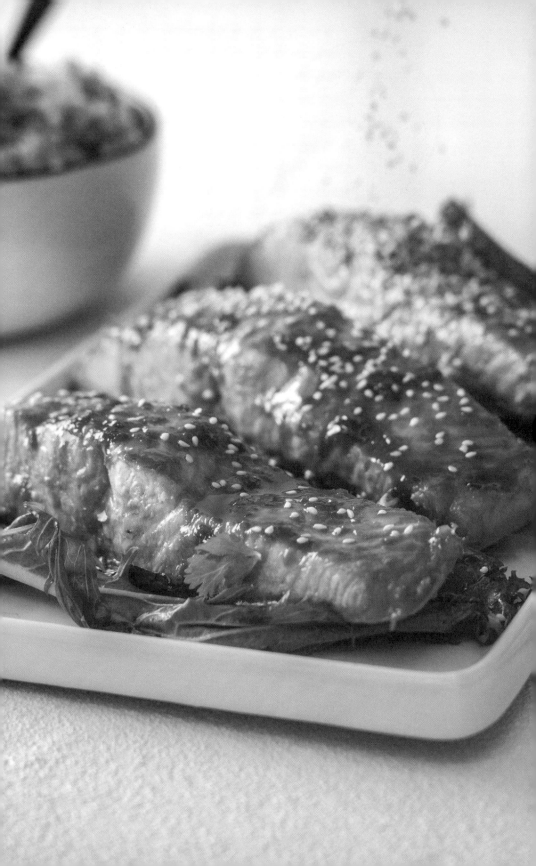

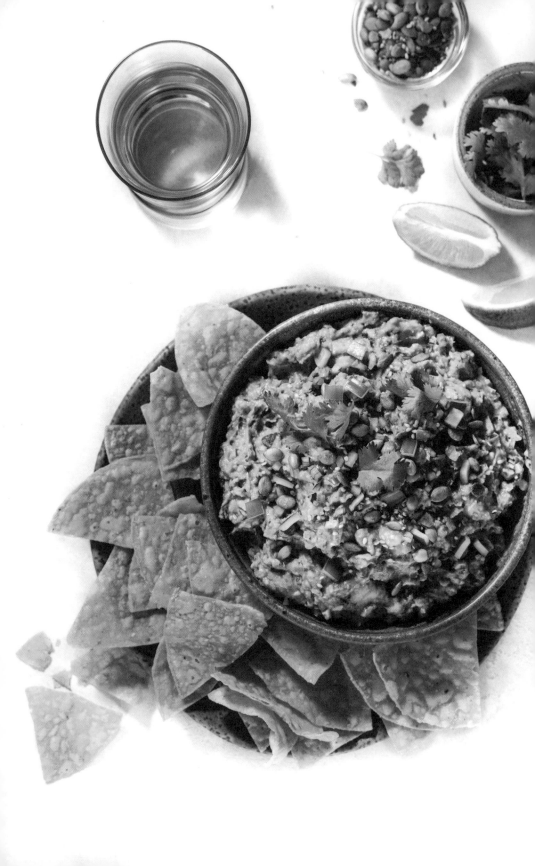

Genius Guacamole with Toasted Seeds

MAKES 4 SERVINGS

Combining seeds with avocado brings our favorite dip to a whole new brain-boosting level! Avocado improves blood flow and oxygenation, while pumpkin, hemp, and sesame seeds contain B vitamins and omega-3s, which have both been shown to slow the rate of cognitive decline. Mix these superstars together, serve with a rainbow of sliced veggies (more brain food), and get ready for enhanced concentration and a longer attention span.

Tip: Store any uneaten guacamole with the avocado pit in the bowl to prevent browning.

INGREDIENTS

2 Tbsp pumpkin seeds

1 Tbsp sesame seeds

1 Tbsp hemp seeds

3 or 4 large ripe avocados (about 1¼ lbs), pitted, peeled, and cut into chunks

2 Tbsp fresh lime juice, plus more as needed

½ tsp ground cumin

½ tsp fine sea salt, plus more to taste

¼ cup chopped fresh cilantro, plus more for garnish

3 Tbsp finely chopped red onion

½ medium jalapeño, seeded and minced

1 garlic clove, minced

Pinch of crushed red pepper flakes

Tortilla chips and/or sliced vegetables, such as carrot sticks, bell pepper strips, jicama, or celery, for serving

1. In a medium frying pan over medium heat, toast the pumpkin, sesame, and hemp seeds, stirring occasionally, until fragrant and golden brown, 2 to 3 minutes. Transfer to a bowl and let cool completely.

2. In a medium bowl using a fork, mash together the avocado, lime juice, cumin, and salt, leaving the mixture slightly chunky. Stir in the cilantro, onion, jalapeño, and garlic until well combined. Sprinkle with the crushed red pepper flakes, then season with additional salt and lime juice if needed.

3. Transfer to a shallow serving bowl. Garnish with the toasted seeds, cilantro, and a squeeze of lime. Serve immediately with chips and/or veggies.

Chocolate-Pistachio Bark with Freeze-Dried Raspberries

MAKES ABOUT 20 3-INCH PIECES

Ready for another reason to eat chocolate? It's a fermented food that can increase beneficial bacteria and strengthen the connection between the gut and the brain. Cacao is also high in flavonols, proven to improve blood flow to the brain. Adding healthy fats from the nuts plus antioxidants from the berries and zest transforms these ingredients into a mouthwatering focus-food treat. Refer back to the Chocolate Meditation (page 98) to get the most satisfaction from this bark!

Tip: Other topping combo ideas include dried blueberries and hemp seeds, goji berries and slivered almonds, dried apricots and pumpkin seeds, and dried figs and walnuts.

INGREDIENTS

1 lb dark chocolate (70 percent cacao or higher)

1 cup (1 oz) freeze-dried raspberries, roughly crushed

1 cup (4 oz) roasted pistachios, roughly chopped

2 tsp finely grated orange zest (optional)

1 tsp flaky sea salt, or to taste (optional)

1. Line a large rimmed baking sheet with parchment paper. In a heatproof bowl set over a pan of barely simmering water (not touching the water), melt the chocolate, stirring until smooth.

2. Remove the chocolate from the heat. Stir in half of the freeze-dried raspberries and half of the chopped pistachios until well combined.

3. Pour the chocolate mixture onto the parchment. Using a thin metal spatula, spread the mixture into a thin rectangle that measures about 10 by 15 inches. Working quickly, sprinkle the remaining freeze-dried raspberries and pistachios evenly over the chocolate, add the orange zest, then sprinkle with the flaky salt, adding more if you like.

4. Refrigerate, uncovered, until set, about 1 hour. Chop or break into pieces to serve. Store leftovers in an airtight container at room temperature for up to 1 week.

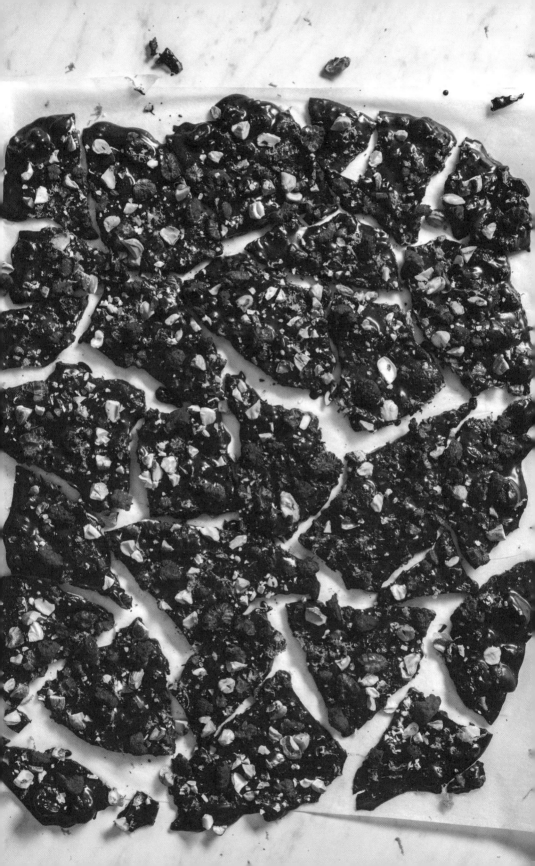

Elise's Brain-Boosting Matcha Latte

MAKES 1 SERVING

Create a grounding ritual with an antioxidant-rich matcha latte. Double the brain-boosting benefits with the nutrients in this pure form of green tea by taking a few minutes to slowly sip and breathe. Not only does savoring what you're drinking allow your mind to relax, it also provides an opportunity for you to slow down, think more clearly, and just be. Matcha contains L-theanine, an amino acid that promotes alpha-wave brain production (similar to what you experience when you meditate), which results in a steady boost in energy and focus without the typical crash of caffeine.

Tip: After years of experimentation, this combination is my tried-and-true recipe to stay sharp and focused. MCT oil (often referred to as brain fuel) helps with absorption of nutrients, and tocos (short for the vitamin E derivative tocotrienols) makes the latte extra creamy with a side of beautifying skin food.

INGREDIENTS

1 tsp matcha tea

¼ to ½ cup hot (not boiling) water

¾ cup plant-based milk (I love oat or coconut milk in this recipe)

1 to 2 tsp tocos

1 tsp MCT oil

maple syrup or sweetener of choice, to taste

1. Add the matcha tea to a large mug or matcha bowl. Mix in the hot water and whisk until well combined and any clumps have dissipated. In a small saucepan over low heat, gently warm the milk until steaming.

2. Transfer the milk and matcha mixture to a blender (or use a handheld frother). Add the tocos, MCT oil, and maple syrup to sweeten as desired.

3. Blend until well combined and the latte is foamy, 20 to 30 seconds. Pour the mixture back to the mug or matcha bowl. Sip and enjoy!

FOCUSED FOOD-MOOD CHEAT SHEET

Quick tip: Choose healthy fats to improve cognitive functions and magnesium-rich foods to ease stress.

avocado
broccoli
cinnamon
eggs
fatty fish and shellfish
fermented foods (such
  as kimchi, tempeh,
  miso, sauerkraut)
garlic
ginger
herbs (such as oregano,
  rosemary, thyme,
  lemon balm)

leafy greens
matcha tea
MCT oil
nuts (especially
  walnuts)
seeds
turmeric
yogurt (dairy or
  non-dairy)

FOCUSED RITUAL

Strengthen Your Attention!

Just as athletes take recovery days and many religions require a day of rest, our brains need down time to reset and recover in order to keep functioning at their best. Meals are the optimal time to take a break. To reduce overwhelm and be better able to focus on the food in front of you, start a practice of minimizing distractions that are coming from your overthinking mind.

Grab a piece of paper or open up the notes section on your phone, then just release all the thoughts that are buzzing around inside. Your long to-do lists. Your upcoming events. Laundry. Groceries. Meal prep. Things you don't want to forget. Write them all down. You can do this before you turn to anything that requires focus, not just meals. Do it when you're going to write, study, cook, attend a meeting, whenever! It's like a giant brain dump to clear your head.

Try this ritual once a day and notice how much more present and attentive you feel. Ideally, you'll turn this practice into a habit whenever you observe your attention drifting in many different directions.

RADIANT

Iced Raspberry Rose Latte

Rosewater has been used as a beautifying ingredient since the time of Cleopatra. Take a modern approach by infusing your nut milk with antioxidant-rich raspberries plus the feel-good and antiaging properties of rose to get glowing from the inside out. Don't let the simplicity of this latte fool you: despite having only a handful of ingredients, the result is luscious and satisfying.

INGREDIENTS

¾ cup plant-based milk, such as almond or coconut

⅓ cup fresh or frozen raspberries

2 tsp maple syrup or other sweetener, or to taste

½ to 1 tsp rosewater, or to taste

¼ tsp vanilla extract

1. Place all of the ingredients in a blender and blend until the raspberries are puréed and the mixture is well combined, about 30 seconds. Strain through a fine-mesh sieve into a tall glass. Add enough ice to fill the glass and serve.

Eat Pretty Salad

Flood your body with ingredients that help you get that plant-powered gorgeous glow. This colorful, crunchy salad is bursting with skin-boosting nutrients along with flavor and texture. The jicama is high in inulin, a prebiotic fiber that helps to restore good gut bacteria. The beta carotene from the carrots is converted into vitamin A in your body and will leave your complexion looking vibrant and bright. Slightly sweet spiced pecans make it easy to fill up on omega-3s. Then mix in grapefruit wedges and the tangy grapefruit vinaigrette for a big old dose of antiaging vitamins C and E!

SPICED PECANS

½ cup chopped raw pecans

2 tsp maple syrup

1 tsp avocado oil

⅛ tsp ground cinnamon

⅛ tsp fine sea salt

pinch of cayenne pepper

GRAPEFRUIT VINAIGRETTE

3 Tbsp fresh grapefruit juice

2 Tbsp fresh lime juice

1 Tbsp rice wine vinegar

1 tsp reduced-sodium tamari or soy sauce

1 tsp maple syrup

fine sea salt and freshly ground black pepper

¼ cup avocado oil

SALAD

3 cups mixed baby lettuces

1 cup finely shredded red cabbage

about 4 oz jicama, peeled and cut into thin matchsticks

1 carrot, peeled and shredded

1 large grapefruit, peeled

¼ cup loosely packed chopped fresh mint leaves

edible flowers, for garnish (optional)

1. Preheat the oven to 325°F. To make the pecans, in a bowl toss together all of the ingredients until evenly coated. Spread onto a rimmed baking sheet. Roast, stirring occasionally, until the nuts are fragrant and toasted, 10 to 13 minutes. Set aside to cool completely.

2. To make the vinaigrette, in a blender combine the grapefruit juice, lime juice, vinegar, tamari, maple syrup, a pinch of salt, and a few grinds of pepper. Process to combine. With the machine running, slowly add the oil, blending until the vinaigrette is emulsified. Pour into a bowl.

3. In a shallow serving bowl, toss together the lettuces, cabbage, jicama, and shredded carrot. Drizzle with a few tablespoons of vinaigrette and toss to coat evenly.

4. Using a knife, segment the grapefruit and discard any seeds. Add to the vegetables in the serving bowl along with the mint and reserved pecans and toss gently. Drizzle with a little more vinaigrette. Garnish with the edible flowers, if using. Serve, passing the remaining vinaigrette alongside.

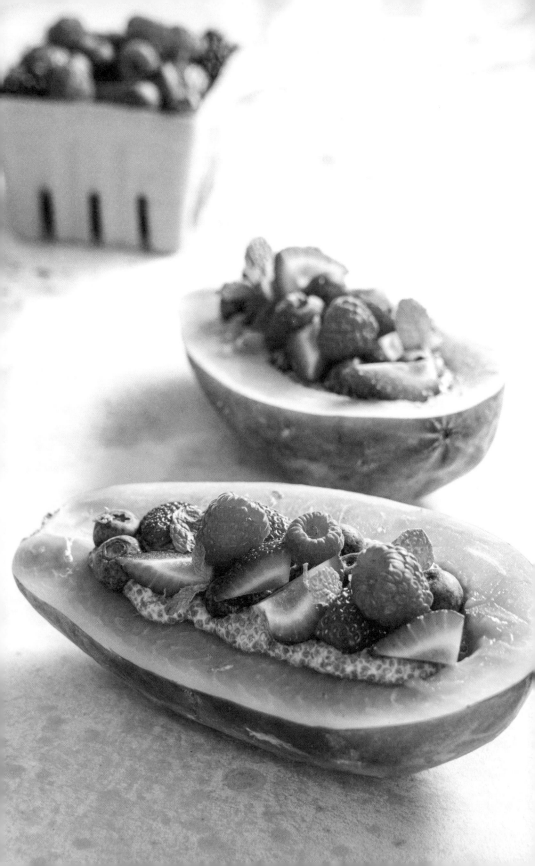

Papaya Boats with Lime Chia Pudding

MAKES 2 SERVINGS

One of the top beauty foods, juicy tropical papayas are packed with nutrients and an abundance of collagen-stimulating vitamin C to keep your skin supple and nourished. For a radiant breakfast or snack, this extra-hydrating fruit serves as an edible bowl filled with creamy, lime-scented chia pudding. Chia seeds—also super hydrating—are loaded with healthy omega-3 fatty acids and protein, both crucial components for synthesizing collagen. Top it off with a squeeze of lime.

INGREDIENTS

1 cup plant-based milk, ideally coconut milk

1 Tbsp maple syrup, or to taste

finely grated zest of 1 lime, plus extra for garnish

½ tsp vanilla extract

pinch of fine sea salt

¼ cup chia seeds

1 medium ripe papaya

1 lime, cut in half

1 cup fresh mixed berries, such as raspberries, blueberries, and blackberries

2 Tbsp roughly chopped fresh mint leaves

1. To make the chia seed pudding, in a bowl combine the milk, maple syrup, lime zest, vanilla, and salt. Whisk to blend. Add the chia seeds and whisk until well combined. Cover the bowl or transfer to a mason jar (making sure the pudding has room to expand). Refrigerate for at least 3 hours or up to overnight, ideally stirring once after the pudding starts to thicken (after about 2 hours) to help distribute the chia seeds evenly.

2. When ready to eat, slice the papaya in half lengthwise, then scoop out and discard the seeds. Place each papaya half on a plate. Squeeze a half of a lime over each papaya half. Stir the chia pudding, then fill the papaya halves with the pudding, dividing it evenly. Top with the berries and mint leaves. Finely grate a little lime zest over the top of each serving. Grab a spoon and dig in!

Parchment Baked Fish with Herbs, Zucchini, and Cherry Tomatoes

MAKES 4 SERVINGS

Baking in parchment is a simple but elegant way to prepare and serve fish. Also known as cooking *en papillote*, the French technique is a healthy method by which to steam and infuse the fillets with a burst of extra flavor. Plus the parchment "packages" make an impressive presentation. This light dish boasts an abundance of skin-supporting nutrients: the fish provides protein to promote collagen production; tomatoes contain lycopene, a powerful antioxidant that helps protect your skin from sun damage; and anti-inflammatory herbs soothe the appearance of stressed-out skin.

Tip: Choose tender, flaky white fillets, such as petrale sole or flounder. If you like, instead of using spiral-cut zucchini, cut 2 small zucchinis into thin matchsticks. Use any fresh, tender herbs you have on hand.

INGREDIENTS

2 cups spiral-cut zucchini

fine sea salt and freshly ground pepper

4 white fish fillets, such as sole or flounder (each about 6 oz)

1 cup quartered cherry tomatoes

2 Tbsp extra-virgin olive oil

1 Tbsp chopped fresh herbs, such as thyme, oregano, and/or parsley, plus garnish

¼ lemon, plus slices for garnish

1. Preheat the oven to 400°F. Cut four pieces of parchment paper into 12-inch squares.

2. Divide the zucchini between the parchment pieces, placing it in the center of each square. Season with a little salt. Top each zucchini pile with a fish fillet. Season fillets lightly with salt and pepper. Scatter the cherry tomatoes over the fish fillets, dividing evenly. Drizzle each portion with the oil and sprinkle with the herbs. Squeeze the juice from the lemon over the top.

3. Lift the two longer sides of the parchment paper to meet in the middle above each fish fillet. Tightly roll the paper down to meet the fish, then crimp and roll the ends, tucking them underneath the package to seal.

4. Place the parchment packages on a baking sheet in a single layer. Bake until the fish is cooked through and the vegetables are crisp-tender, about 10 minutes for thin fillets or 15 minutes for thicker fillets.

5. Transfer each packet to a plate, unwrap, garnish with fresh herbs and sliced lemon, and serve.

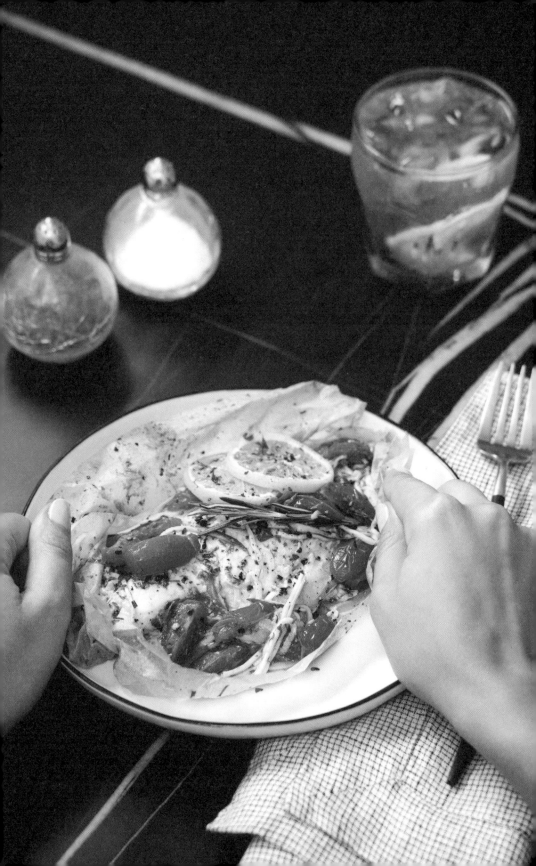

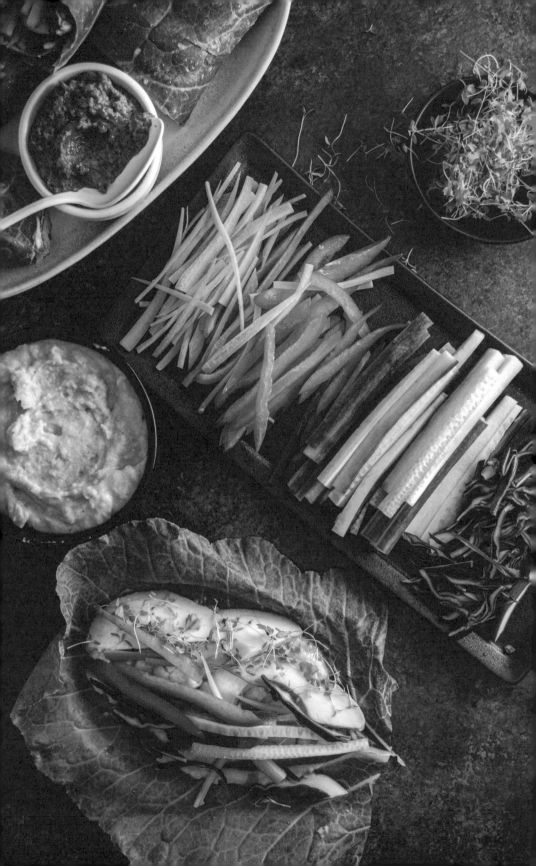

Mediterranean Collard Wraps

MAKES 4 SERVINGS

A rainbow of fresh veggies nestle inside tender collard leaves, creating these bright and colorful wraps. Loaded with collagen-stimulating vitamin C, vibrant vegetables help keep your skin feeling firm and elastic. The velvety white bean spread and tangy, nutty-sweet romesco sauce—both packed with bold anti-inflammatory ingredients and seasonings—elevate these wraps with skin-boosting nutrients and out-of-this world flavors.

Tip: Substitute hummus or sweet potato purée for the white bean purée. Use the romesco sauce as a spread on pita or toast with thick slices of fresh tomatoes, or serve it alongside roasted veggies or grilled fish or chicken.

ROMESCO SAUCE

⅓ cup chopped toasted walnuts or almonds

½ cup chopped roasted red pepper

¼ cup crushed or puréed tomatoes

2 Tbsp fresh flat-leaf Italian parsley

1 Tbsp vinegar, such as sherry, red wine, or balsamic

1 clove garlic, chopped

1 tsp sweet paprika

⅓ cup extra-virgin olive oil

fine sea salt and freshly ground pepper

WHITE BEAN PURÉE

1 Tbsp extra-virgin olive oil

2 cloves garlic, minced

1 15.5-oz can cannellini beans, rinsed and drained (about 1½ cups cooked beans)

¼ cup vegetable broth

fine sea salt and freshly ground pepper

WRAPS

4 large collard leaves

4-inch piece English cucumber, peeled, halved lengthwise, and cut lengthwise into 8 thin pieces

½ red or orange bell pepper, seeded, membranes removed, and thinly sliced lengthwise

1 medium carrot, peeled and shredded (about ½ cup packed)

½ cup packed finely shredded purple cabbage

½ large ripe avocado, pitted, peeled, and thinly sliced

½ cup microgreens

1. For the romesco sauce: In the bowl of a food processor, pulse the nuts to a fine meal. Add the roasted red pepper, tomatoes, parsley, vinegar, garlic, and paprika. With the machine running, drizzle in the olive oil. Transfer to a bowl. Season to taste with salt and pepper.

Mediterranean Collard Wraps (cont.)

2. For the white bean purée: In a small saucepan over medium heat, simmer the olive oil and garlic, stirring, until fragrant, about 1 minute. Add the beans and broth and bring to a gentle boil. Reduce the heat to low and simmer until slightly thickened, 3 to 4 minutes. Transfer the mixture to the clean bowl of the food processor and purée. Scrape into a bowl and season with salt and pepper; the bean purée should be smooth, thick, and spreadable (like hummus).

3. Rinse and dry the collard leaves. Cut out and discard the thick stem to about halfway up the leaf, so the leaf is pliable and can be rolled into a wrap. The leaf should be about 8 inches wide and 9 to 10 inches long.

4. For each wrap: Spread ¼ cup white bean purée across the bottom third of the leaf (where you removed the stem), spreading an area about 3 inches wide and leaving about 2 inches clear at the bottom and 1 inch clear on either outer edge. Layer the veggies in a row on top of the bean purée in this order: 2 slices cucumber, 4 to 6 slices bell pepper, 2 tablespoons each shredded carrot and shredded cabbage, a quarter of the avocado slices, and 2 tablespoons microgreens.

5. Fold the outer edges of the leaf inward, then fold the bottom of the leaf up and over the ingredients. Roll up as you would a burrito, folding in the edges as you roll and keeping the wrap nice and tight. (Be careful not to let the leaf tear.) Cut the roll into two halves. Serve with the romesco sauce for dipping.

RADIANT FOOD-MOOD CHEAT SHEET

Quick tip: Choose foods rich in vitamin C and protein, which stimulate collagen production. Healthy fats and high-water-content foods are essential, too.

avocado	lentils
bell peppers	melon
berries	pineapple
carrots	papaya
chia seeds	pomegranates
citrus fruits	rosewater
fish	sweet potatoes
jicama	walnuts
leafy greens	

RADIANT RITUAL

Bask in the Sun!

If you practice yoga, you've probably done plenty of Sun Salutations during class. But have you ever tried these . . . outside in the actual sun? It's a gorgeous experience that can help you release stress. Even if you don't practice yoga, you can skip the poses and still experience the rejuvenating powers of sunshine and fresh air.

Take your mat outside and do a few simple rounds of deep breathing and movement to greet the day. Move through a few postures and sequences that you're familiar with, like Mountain Pose, Forward Fold, Plank, Cobra, Upward Dog, and Downward Dog, or simply sit still or lie down if that's what your body is requesting today. Take a moment to acknowledge what a privilege it is to have a physical body and be alive. Feel the sunlight on your skin. Imagine the sun is filling you with its radiance, infusing you with golden rays that you'll carry with you for the rest of the day.

STRONG

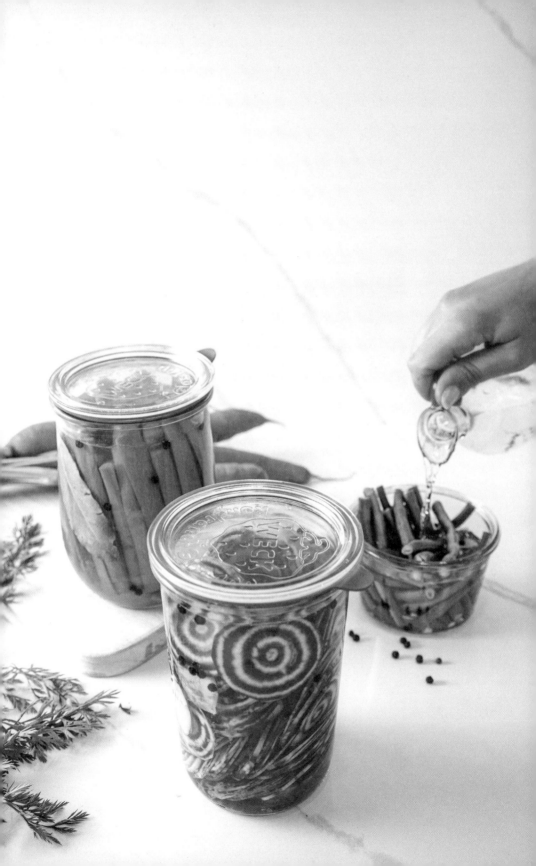

Fermented Veggies

MAKES 4 PINTS

About 80 percent of the immune system resides in the gut, so to feel truly healthy, nourished, and strong, make sure to properly feed yours. Naturally fermented vegetables are packed with an abundance of probiotics and other beneficial bacteria. All you need are a handful of ingredients, plus a little bit of patience, to make your own. Be sure to use distilled, spring, or filtered water and non-iodized salt, or your fermentation will be impeded. For this recipe, you'll need four sterilized pint jars with lids.

INGREDIENTS

about 1 pound red beets

2 bunches small radishes

about ½ pound small carrots

about ½ pound green beans

4 cups distilled water

2 Tbsp fine sea salt or other non-iodized salt

1. Peel the beets, halve them lengthwise, and slice them very thinly (about 1/16 inch thick); alternatively, cut them into matchsticks. Stack the beets in one of the pint jars.

2. Trim the radishes and cut them in halves or quarters, depending on how large they are, then slice them into 1/8-inch-thick slices. Pack them into one of the pint jars.

3. Trim the carrots and peel or scrub them well. Halve them lengthwise or cut them into sticks; they should come no further than about 1 inch below the rim of a pint jar. Pack them into one of the jars.

4. Trim the green beans so they come no further than about 1 inch below the rim of a pint jar. Tightly pack them into the jar.

5. In a large glass measuring pitcher or a bowl, stir together the water and salt until the salt dissolves. Pour the salt water over the vegetables, leaving at least 1 inch of space at the top of the jar. Cover the jars tightly and set aside at room temperature. Once a day, open each jar to release the gases produced during fermentation. If any mold or scum forms on top, skim it off. Taste the fermented vegetables, and when they are done to your liking (usually after 3 to 5 days), transfer them to the refrigerator; chilling will slow down the fermentation. Store in the refrigerator for up to 1 month.

FLAVORING VARIATIONS

Optional ideas to add aromatics and spices:

- Beets with 3 slices fresh ginger and ½ teaspoon orange zest
- Carrots with 1 bay leaf and 1 teaspoon coriander seeds
- Green beans with 1 or 2 sprigs fresh dill and 1 teaspoon mustard seeds
- Radishes with 1 sliced clove garlic

Rainbow Sushi Rolls

MAKES 4 SERVINGS

The easiest way to inundate your body with nutrients and phytonutrients—the healthy chemicals produced by plants—is to eat the rainbow. You don't need to count or measure or follow a list of food rules. Just load up your plate with vibrant, bold hues, and you are well on your way to health. These homemade sushi rolls are just the ticket for getting a variety of bright colors.

Making sushi might sound like a daunting task, but it's actually a fun activity the entire family can enjoy, and most of the ingredients can be prepped in advance. Mix and match the fillings or use quick-pickled daikon radish and carrot, asparagus, cucumber, and creamy avocado. Once you get the method down, it's easy to personalize and make them your own.

Tip: Try lightly cooked shiitake mushrooms, cooked sweet potato spears, marinated tofu strips, bell pepper, and/or smoked salmon for variety.

QUICK PICKLED VEGGIES

3 Tbsp unseasoned rice vinegar

1 tsp coconut sugar

1 small daikon radish (2 oz), peeled and cut into thin matchsticks

1 small carrot (2 oz), peeled and cut into thin matchsticks

SUSHI ROLLS

12 medium-thin asparagus spears, snapped

7-inch piece English cucumber, peeled

4 nori (seaweed sheets)

1 ripe avocado, pitted, peeled, and quartered

tamari or soy sauce, pickled ginger, and/or wasabi, for serving (optional)

SUSHI RICE

1 cup short-grain brown rice

½ tsp fine sea salt

3 Tbsp unseasoned rice vinegar

1 Tbsp coconut sugar

1. To make the pickled veggies, in a small saucepan warm the vinegar and sugar over medium heat, stirring until the sugar dissolves. Add the daikon and carrot to a bowl and pour the vinegar mixture over the vegetables. Stir to combine and set aside at room temperature to cool. Stir every so often.

2. To make the sushi rice, in a medium saucepan stir together the rice, 1¾ cups water, and the salt. Bring to a boil over high heat, then reduce the heat to low, cover, and cook until the rice is tender and the water is absorbed, about 45 minutes. While the rice cooks, in a small saucepan warm the vinegar and sugar over medium heat, stirring until the sugar dissolves. Set aside to cool. Remove the rice from the heat and leave covered and undisturbed for 10 minutes. Using a fork, stir in the vinegar mixture. Let sit, uncovered, until the rice absorbs the vinegar mixture. It should be sticky and dry.

3. Bring a saucepan half-full of lightly salted water to a boil over high heat. Add the asparagus and cook just until crisp-tender, about 1 minute. Drain and rinse under cold water to stop the cooking. Transfer to paper towels and dry well. Halve the cucumber lengthwise. Reserve one half for another use. Scoop out and discard the seeds of the other half using a small spoon. Slice lengthwise into 8 equal strips.

4. Place a bamboo sushi mat on a work surface and cover with a piece of plastic wrap or parchment paper. Lay one piece of nori on top, rough side up and shiny side down, arranging it with the shorter edge closest to you. Scoop a quarter of the cooked rice onto the nori. Using damp hands, spread the rice into a thin, even layer, leaving about 1 inch empty at the top of the nori.

5. Placing the vegetables crosswise across the rice about 1½ inches up from the bottom, neatly arrange 2 strips of cucumber, 3 asparagus spears, and a quarter of the pickled carrot and daikon. Thinly slice a quarter of the avocado and lay the slices across the top of the vegetables. Fold the bottom edge of the rice-covered nori up and over the vegetables, using the mat and plastic wrap to help you compress it down and into itself, until you have rolled it up completely. Brush a little water along the inside top edge and seal the edge. Repeat with the remaining ingredients to create 4 rolls.

6. To serve, cut each sushi roll into 6 to 8 pieces. Arrange on a plate alongside small bowls of tamari with some pickled ginger and wasabi, if desired. Enjoy!

Roasted Whole Cauliflower with Indian Spices and Cilantro Chutney

MAKES 4 SERVINGS AS A MAIN OR 6 SERVINGS AS A SIDE

An entire head of roasted cauliflower is always impressive and makes a gorgeous centerpiece for a meal. Here, the cauliflower is rubbed with an Indian-inspired spice paste and roasted until golden brown and tender, then served with a bright, spicy cilantro chutney. It is utterly delicious! While cauliflower, a cruciferous vegetable naturally high in cancer-fighting compounds and fiber (among many other nutrients), takes center stage here, the real stars are the anti-inflammatory spices in the paste and sauce. The chutney is made with cilantro, a powerful herb that can rid the body of free radicals, detoxify heavy metals, and even lower anxiety.

ROASTED CAULIFLOWER

2 Tbsp melted coconut oil or avocado oil

2 cloves garlic, minced

1 tsp fine sea salt

1 tsp ground cumin

½ tsp ground coriander

½ tsp ground turmeric

½ tsp ground ancho chili powder

¼ tsp ground ginger

1 head cauliflower (about 1½ lbs)

CILANTRO CHUTNEY

1½ cups packed, roughly chopped fresh cilantro (leaves and tender stems)

2 green onions, roughly chopped

1 small jalapeño, seeded and chopped

juice of ½ lime or lemon, plus more if needed

1 Tbsp avocado oil

1 tsp coconut sugar or maple syrup (optional)

½ tsp cumin

¼ tsp coriander

¼ tsp fine sea salt

1. Preheat the oven to 400°F. Place a 10-inch cast-iron pan on the middle rack in the oven. Place another small heatproof pan three-quarters full of water in the bottom of the oven. (This helps create steam.)

2. In a bowl, whisk together the oil, garlic, salt, and spices. Set aside. Rinse and dry the head of cauliflower. On a cutting board, turn the cauliflower head upside down and trim away the large leaves at the bottom. Carefully cut out the base of the core, leaving the florets attached and the head intact. Trim away any remaining leaves.

3. Brush the underside of the cauliflower with about one-third of the spice paste. Turn the cauliflower right-side up and brush the remaining spice paste all over, making sure to get it into as many nooks and crannies as you can.

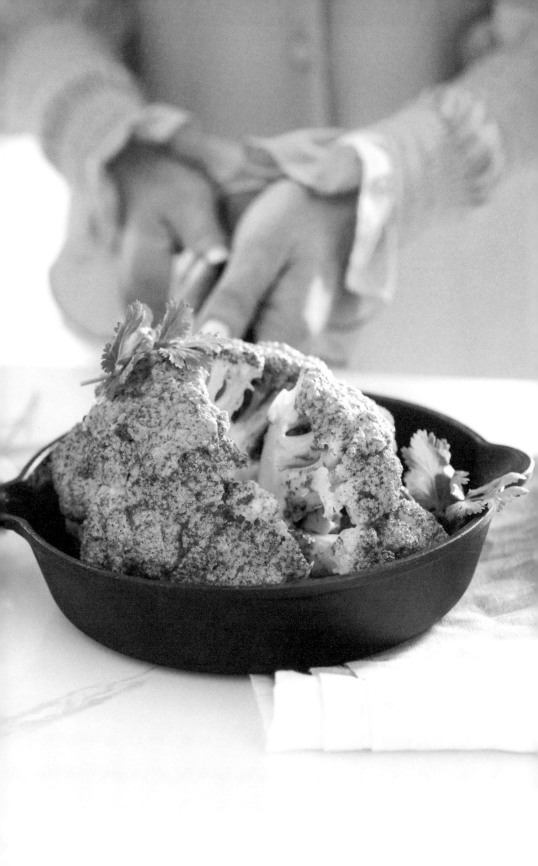

Roasted Whole Cauliflower (cont.)

4. Transfer the cauliflower to the hot cast-iron pan, placing it right-side up. Roast until a knife easily pierces the core and the cauliflower is nicely browned and tender, 45 to 50 minutes. (The timing also depends on whether you like your cauliflower crisp-tender or softer.)

5. While the cauliflower roasts, make the chutney. In a blender, combine the cilantro, green onion, jalapeño, lime or lemon juice, oil, coconut sugar or maple syrup (if using), cumin, coriander, salt, and 2 tablespoons water. Blend until smooth, adding a little more water if needed to create a smooth sauce. Taste and adjust the seasoning with salt, lime or lemon juice, and/or coconut sugar.

6. Transfer the cauliflower to a cutting board and cut into wedges. Serve wedges with the chutney drizzled over the top.

Thai Veggie Curry

MAKES 4 SERVINGS

This Thai-inspired red curry is packed with potent anti-inflammatory spices that help protect your body on a cellular level and keep you feeling healthy and—you guessed it—strong! Feel free to substitute other vegetables or use more (or less) of whatever you have on hand.

Tip: For more protein, add cubed tofu or cooked chicken to the curry mixture and simmer until warmed through, about 10 minutes.

INGREDIENTS

1 cup small broccoli florets

1 cup green beans, cut into 1½-inch lengths

3 Tbsp Thai red curry paste

2 Tbsp coconut aminos

finely grated zest of ½ lime

juice of 1 lime, or to taste

2 Tbsp coconut or avocado oil

½ small yellow onion, finely chopped

fine sea salt

½ large red bell pepper, seeded and sliced

2 medium carrots, peeled and cut into thin matchsticks

2 cloves garlic, minced

1 tsp peeled and grated fresh ginger

1 13.5-oz can coconut milk

3 Makrut lime leaves (optional)

1 cup sugar snap peas, cut into ½-inch pieces on the diagonal

steamed brown rice and lime wedges, for serving

1. Bring a small saucepan half-full of lightly salted water to a boil, then blanch the broccoli until crisp-tender, 1 to 2 minutes. Use a slotted spoon to transfer the broccoli to a colander set in the sink. Bring the water back to a boil, then add the green beans. Blanch until crisp-tender, 1 to 2 minutes. Drain in the colander with the broccoli, then rinse the vegetables in cold water until cool. Set aside.

2. In a small bowl, whisk together the curry paste, coconut aminos, lime zest, and lime juice.

3. In a deep sauté pan over medium heat, warm 1 tablespoon oil. Add the onion and a pinch of salt and cook until softened, stirring, for about 3 minutes. Add the remaining 1 tablespoon oil, then add the bell pepper, carrots, garlic, and ginger and cook, stirring occasionally, until the vegetables are crisp-tender, about 3 minutes.

4. Add the curry mixture to the vegetables along with the coconut milk and lime leaves, if using. Add the sugar snap peas and reserved broccoli and green beans to the pan. Bring to a simmer, then reduce the heat to low and simmer gently until the vegetables are tender, about 5 minutes.

5. To serve, remove the lime leaves. Spoon rice into 4 shallow bowls and ladle the curry over the top. Squeeze a wedge of lime over each bowl. Serve warm.

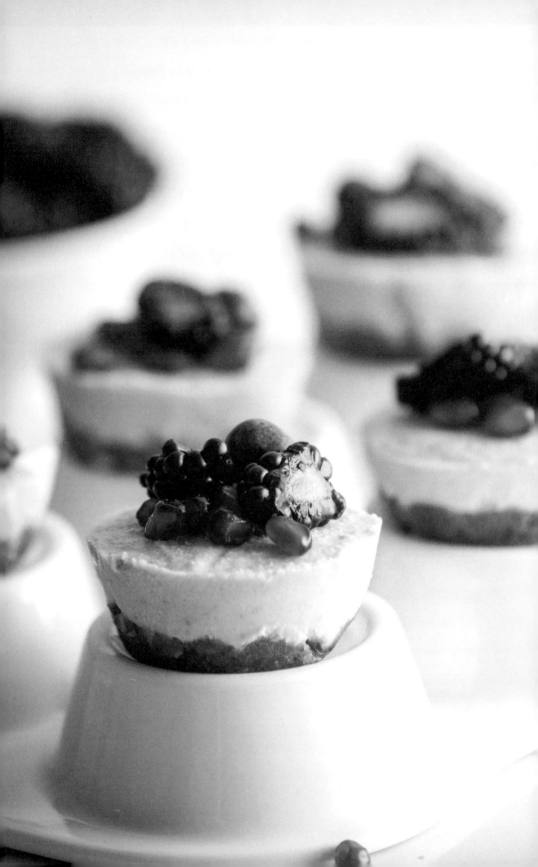

Vegan Cashew Cheesecakes with Purple Fruit

MAKES 12 MINI CHEESECAKES

You would never believe that these ultracreamy cheesecakes are completely vegan and gluten free! The decadent vanilla filling is made with soaked cashews blended with coconut milk and maple syrup. You can use any fruit that is fragrant, ripe, and in season, but the darker the fruit, the higher the antioxidant level. That's why I love using purple-pigmented blackberries, plums, and blueberries. These fruits contain flavonoids, including resveratrol, which can help boost overall immunity and protect against certain cancers.

Tip: For the crust, process toasted walnuts or pecans in a food processor to a fine meal and use an equal amount in place of the almond flour.

CRUST

1 cup chopped pitted Medjool dates (about 6.5 oz)

½ cup almond flour

¼ cup unsweetened shredded coconut

¼ tsp vanilla extract

⅛ tsp fine sea salt

PURPLE FRUIT

about 3 cups chopped fresh purple fruit, cut into bite-sized pieces, such as plums, blueberries, and blackberries

2 Tbsp maple syrup or coconut sugar, or to taste (optional)

VANILLA CASHEW FILLING

1½ cups (½ lb) raw cashews

½ cup coconut milk

⅓ cup maple syrup

¼ cup coconut oil, melted

3 Tbsp fresh lemon juice

1 tsp vanilla extract

⅛ tsp fine sea salt

1. Cover the cashews in cold water and soak for at least 4 hours or up to overnight; alternatively, soak them in hot water for 15 minutes.

2. Grease a standard 12-cup muffin pan. Cut 12 strips of parchment paper that are each about 7 inches long and lay them into the 12 muffin cups so the ends come up and over two of the sides. (This will make removing the cheesecakes easier.)

3. To make the crust, in the bowl of a food processor, process the dates until very finely chopped and the mixture balls up. Add the almond flour, coconut, vanilla, and salt and process until well combined; the mixture should be crumbly but hold together when pressed between your fingers. Scoop about 1½ tablespoons of the crust mixture into each muffin cup.

Vegan Cashew Cheesecakes (cont.)

Using your fingers or the bottom of a small glass, press the mixture into a solid, even layer covering the bottom of each cup. Set the pan in the freezer while you make the filling.

4. Drain the cashews and add to a blender, then add the remaining filling ingredients. Blend on high speed until the mixture is very smooth and silky, about 2 minutes.

5. Divide the filling evenly between the muffin cups. Tap down the pan on the work surface to remove any air pockets. Cover and freeze until firm, at least 3 hours. To remove, run a knife around the edge to help loosen the cheesecakes, then pull up the parchment tabs.

6. In a bowl, toss the fruit together with the maple syrup or coconut sugar, if using. To serve, top each cheesecake with a big spoonful of the fruit (about ¼ cup). The cheesecakes can be served frozen, or let them soften slightly at room temperature before serving. (The cheesecakes will keep for up to 2 weeks in the freezer.)

STRONG FOOD-MOOD CHEAT SHEET

Quick tip: Choose foods straight from the earth and let the farmers' market become your pharmacy. Plant medicine is powerful—with tasty and delicious benefits.

berries
cilantro
elderberry extract
fermented foods
garlic
ginger
herbs (such as cilantro, parsley, oregano, rosemary, holy basil)

honey (raw)
leafy greens
lemon
matcha tea
mushrooms
probiotic-rich foods
turmeric

STRONG RITUAL

Shift Your Surroundings, Feel Your Power Grow!

Take a look at your dining area, bedroom, office, or any place where you spend a lot of time. How is the furniture arranged? How do you feel being in this space? Powerful? In charge? Or vaguely unsettled, anxious, and threatened?

We instinctively feel secure, powerful, and strong when sitting and sleeping in positions where we can see the room's doorway and with a solid wall behind us. Consider moving your desk, bed, and other furniture so that you have a clear view of your surroundings and can assume what's called the command position in feng shui. See how it feels. You might notice an immediate shift!

And if you think feng shui is just woo-woo nonsense, think again. There's an entire branch of social science called environmental psychology that studies how our physical surroundings influence our mental and physical health. Turns out, the positioning of your furniture really *does* impact your stress levels and immune system. Who knew that rearranging the couch could help you fight off a cold?

COMFORTED

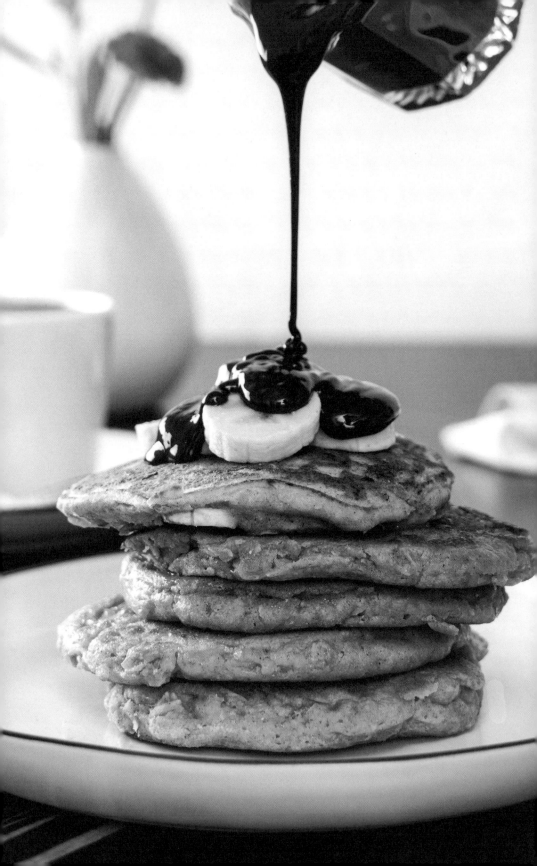

Oaty Pancakes with Banana Coins

MAKES 4 TO 6 SERVINGS

Pancakes are one of those breakfast dishes that make you want to jump out of bed, bringing on all sorts of feel-good memories. These fluffy gluten-free pancakes are just the ticket for a trip down memory lane. Cinnamon adds warmth to bring on those cozy vibes, and smashed bananas naturally sweeten the stack while adding a dose of potassium, a natural muscle relaxant.

INGREDIENTS

1 cup oat flour

½ cup brown rice flour

⅓ cup old-fashioned rolled oats

2 tsp baking powder

½ tsp fine sea salt

½ tsp ground cinnamon

¼ tsp ground nutmeg

3 small bananas (ripe but not too brown)

2 large eggs

¾ cup plant-based milk, plus more if needed

2 Tbsp melted coconut oil, plus more for cooking

½ tsp vanilla extract

butter of choice, for serving (optional)

maple syrup, for serving (optional)

melted chocolate, for drizzling (optional but highly recommended)

1. In a medium bowl, whisk together the oat flour, rice flour, oats, baking powder, salt, and spices. In a small mixing bowl, using the back of a fork, mash one banana to a smooth purée. Add the eggs, milk, coconut oil, and vanilla and whisk to combine.

2. Add the wet ingredients to the dry ingredients and stir with a whisk to combine. Let the batter sit for about 10 minutes. If the batter becomes overly thick, add a splash more of the milk. Slice the remaining two bananas into thin, coin-shaped slices.

3. Heat a large skillet or griddle over medium heat. Brush with coconut oil. When the pan and oil are hot, dollop a heaping ¼ cup of the batter into the pan, spreading it evenly into a 4-inch round; you should be able to get 2 to 3 pancakes into the pan, depending on the size of your pan. Add 4 to 6 banana slices in an even layer to the top of each pancake.

4. Cook until the pancakes puff and the undersides are golden, about 2 minutes. Using a spatula, flip the pancakes and continue to cook until they are golden brown and cooked through, about 2 minutes longer. Adjust the heat as needed.

5. Serve warm with your butter of choice, maple syrup, and melted chocolate if desired. To keep the pancakes warm, transfer to a baking sheet and place in a 200°F oven. (The pancakes can be cooled to room temperature, then frozen in a single layer on a baking sheet; pack them in an airtight container separated by parchment paper. To serve, bring to room temperature and reheat in a pan over low heat.)

Homemade Nut Butter and Raspberry Chia Jam on Toasts

MAKES 2 SERVINGS, PLUS LEFTOVER NUT BUTTER AND JAM

PB and Js always make me feel like a kid again. The cacao nibs in the nut butter and chia seeds in the jam give this classic dish a grown-up twist. Aside from creating nostalgic feelings, the nutritionally dense ingredients earn these toasts the title of superfood. Cacao has one of the highest levels of antioxidants of almost any food and also contains anandamide, the bliss molecule, while chia seeds boast mood-balancing omega-3s. Just make sure to spread extra thick layers on your open-faced sandwich. Satisfaction guaranteed!

Tip: The nut butter turns out extra creamy with amazing flavor when the nuts are lightly roasted before processing.

SUPERFOOD NUT BUTTER

1 cup raw cashews

1 cup raw walnuts or pecans

2 Tbsp cacao nibs

1 Tbsp flax meal

1 Tbsp coconut oil

2 tsp maple syrup (optional)

1 tsp ground cinnamon

¼ tsp fine sea salt

2 to 4 slices of your favorite regular or gluten-free bread, toasted (I use sprouted or sourdough bread)

RASPBERRY CHIA JAM

2 cups (10 oz) fresh or thawed frozen raspberries

2 Tbsp maple syrup or honey, or to taste

1 tsp finely grated lemon zest, orange zest, or vanilla extract

1 tsp lemon juice

pinch of fine sea salt

2 Tbsp chia seeds

toppings: fresh berries, hemp seeds, shredded coconut, and/or extra cacao nibs

1. To make the nut butter, preheat the oven to 350°F. Line a rimmed baking sheet with parchment paper. Combine the nuts on the baking sheet and spread into a single layer. Roast until fragrant and golden brown, stirring once halfway through, about 10 minutes. Set aside to cool for about 10 minutes.

2. Transfer the nuts to the bowl of a food processor and process until smooth and creamy, scraping down the sides as necessary, 4 to 6 minutes. Add the cacao nibs, flax meal, coconut oil, maple syrup (if using), cinnamon, and salt. Process until the ingredients are well incorporated and the mixture is smooth with small chunks of cacao nibs visible, about 1 minute. Store in a glass jar at room temperature for up to 1 week or in the refrigerator for up to 3 weeks.

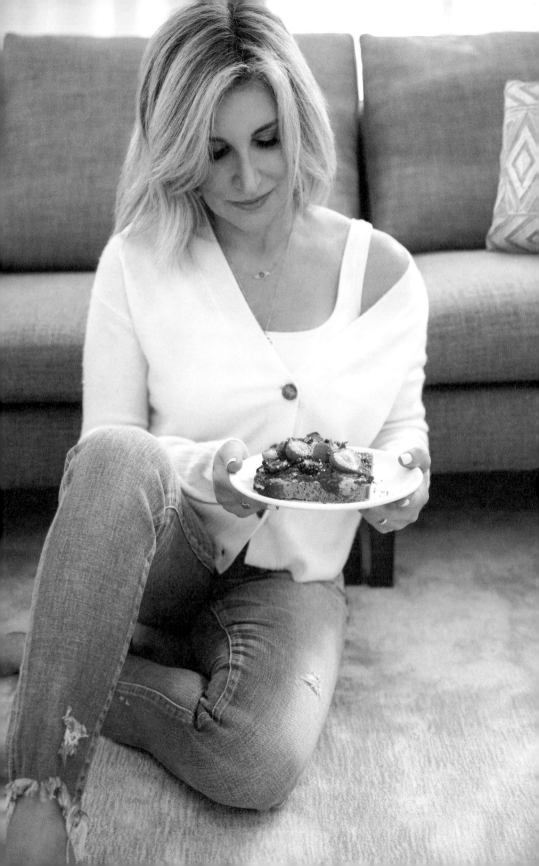

Nut Butter and Jam on Toasts (cont.)

3. To make the jam, in a saucepan mash the raspberries with a fork. If using fresh berries, add ¼ cup water after mashing. Stir in the maple syrup or honey. Bring to a boil over high heat, then reduce to medium-low and simmer, stirring frequently, until the color deepens and the berries start to thicken slightly, about 5 minutes. Remove from the heat and stir in the zest or extract, lemon juice, and salt. Stir in the chia seeds. Set aside to cool completely. Transfer to a glass jar or an airtight container and refrigerate for at least 1 hour before serving. Any remaining jam can be stored in the refrigerator for up to 1 week.

4. Spread each piece of toast with the nut butter, then with the jam. Add toppings of choice, then enjoy your elevated PB and J!

Vegan Mac and Cheese with Creamy Butternut Squash Sauce

MAKES 6 SERVINGS

Mac and cheese is the ultimate comfort food, but this one has a healthy twist: the rich, flavorful sauce is made with butternut squash, cashews, and anti-inflammatory turmeric and garlic. The addition of nutritional yeast gives it a cheesy flavor while keeping it entirely plant based. Use regular or gluten-free pasta and cook only until just barely al dente; you will add it back to the sauce and cook a few extra minutes to warm it through. It's worth the wait!

Tip: For a variation, once you mix the sauce and pasta, transfer the mixture to a greased baking dish, top with panko or bread crumbs, and bake in a 375°F oven until golden, about 20 minutes.

INGREDIENTS

¾ cup raw cashews

2 cups (10 oz) ½-inch cubes butternut squash

1 Tbsp extra-virgin olive oil

½ yellow onion, finely chopped

fine sea salt and freshly ground black pepper

1 clove garlic, minced

2 Tbsp lemon juice, or to taste

1 Tbsp nutritional yeast, or to taste (optional)

2 tsp apple cider vinegar, or to taste

1 tsp turmeric

1 tsp paprika

½ tsp onion powder

½ tsp Dijon mustard

1 lb elbow macaroni (regular, gluten free, or grain free)

1. Cover the cashews in cold water and soak for 2 to 4 hours; alternatively, soak them in hot water for 15 minutes. Drain and add to a blender.

2. In a medium saucepan, combine the cubed butternut squash and 3 cups of water. Bring to a boil over high heat, then reduce the heat to medium-low, partially cover, and simmer, stirring occasionally, until the squash is very tender, about 20 minutes. Drain through a fine-mesh sieve placed over a bowl, reserving the cooking water. Transfer the squash to the blender.

3. Add the oil to the saucepan and warm over medium-low heat. Add the onion and a sprinkle of salt and cook, stirring, until tender and golden, about 5 minutes. Add the garlic and cook until fragrant, about 1 minute. Transfer the onion and garlic to the blender.

4. Add the lemon juice, optional nutritional yeast, vinegar, turmeric, paprika, onion powder, Dijon mustard, ½ teaspoon salt, and ¼ teaspoon pepper

Vegan Mac and Cheese (cont.)

to the blender along with 1½ cups of the reserved squash cooking water. Blend until very creamy, adding hot water as needed to thin to a sauce-like consistency. You'll want it to be a little thinner than desired for serving, as it will thicken slightly once mixed with the pasta.

5. Fill the saucepan half-full of salted water and bring to a boil over high heat. Add the pasta, stir, and reduce the heat to medium-high. Boil until the pasta is al dente, 5 to 7 minutes or according to package directions. Drain and set aside.

6. Transfer the sauce to the saucepan over low heat. Taste and season with additional salt, pepper, lemon juice, nutritional yeast, and/or vinegar to get to the flavor you like. Add the pasta to the sauce and stir to combine; it may seem too thin at first but will thicken as you mix it and it cools slightly. Gently warm the mac and cheese until hot. Serve immediately. (The mac and cheese can be cooled and stored in an airtight container in the refrigerator for up to 5 days. Thin with some water when reheating.)

Cozy Veggie Chili

This veggie-filled chili is a family favorite—it nourishes your body and uplifts your soul. The combination of warming anti-inflammatory spices and hearty beans feels like a cozy hug from the inside out. Peppers, carrots, corn, and tomatoes add both flavor and nutrients. You can mix and match with whatever beans you like: try swapping black beans for garbanzo beans or use all pinto beans. The recipe makes quite a bit of chili, and it can easily be frozen for meals at the ready.

Tip: Canned or jarred beans are convenient, but I prefer to use dried beans whenever possible. If you go the dried bean route, use 4 to 5 cups of mixed cooked beans.

INGREDIENTS

2 Tbsp extra-virgin olive oil or avocado oil

½ yellow onion, finely chopped

1 small red bell pepper, seeded and finely chopped

½ small green or orange bell pepper, seeded and finely chopped

1 large carrot, peeled and finely chopped

1 small jalapeño, seeded and finely chopped

fine sea salt and freshly ground black pepper

3 Tbsp chili powder

1 tsp ground cumin

½ tsp crushed red pepper flakes, or to taste (optional)

1 15.5-oz can red kidney beans, rinsed and drained

1 15.5-oz can pinto beans, rinsed and drained

1 15.5-oz can black beans, rinsed and drained

1 14.5-oz can fire-roasted diced tomatoes, with juices (1½ cups)

1 cup crushed or puréed tomatoes

½ cup fresh or frozen corn kernels

chopped green onion, chopped avocado, and chopped fresh cilantro, for serving (optional)

1. In a large saucepan over medium heat, warm the oil. Add the onion, bell peppers, carrot, jalapeño, and a big pinch of salt and cook, stirring occasionally, until tender and starting to brown, about 7 minutes. Stir in the chili powder, cumin, and red chili flakes until well mixed and fragrant.

2. Add the beans, tomatoes, and 3/4 cup water. Bring to a boil, reduce the heat to low, and simmer, partially covered, until thickened and fragrant, about 45 minutes. About 10 minutes before the chili is ready, add in the corn kernels.

3. Taste and season with salt and pepper. Serve warm, garnished with green onion, avocado, and cilantro, if you like.

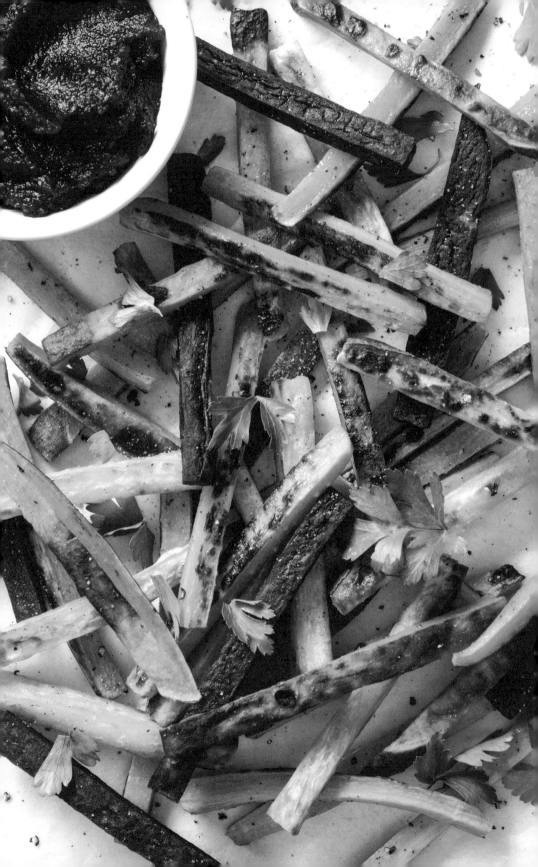

Root Veggie Fries with Beet Ketchup

MAKES 4 SERVINGS

A big bowl of crisp-roasted root veggie fries with a side of homemade ketchup for dipping will bring back all kinds of childhood memories with a grown-up twist. Use sweet potatoes, parsnips, and carrots, or any of your root vegetable favorites. The bold, bright colors of nutrient-dense root vegetables are not just beautiful but also give grounding energy and a boost of serotonin. Be sure to make the beet ketchup, because it is truly mind-blowing and you'll want to eat it with *everything*. It's great spread on a veggie burger and toast with hummus or as a dip for veggies, such as raw celery, raw bell peppers, or crisp-tender roasted asparagus.

Tip: For a more rustic dish, leave the vegetables unpeeled. If you love ketchup, you'll want to double the recipe.

ROOT VEGGIE FRIES

1 medium sweet potato (8 oz)

3 medium carrots (6 oz)

2 medium parsnips (6 oz)

2 Tbsp olive oil or avocado oil

2 Tbsp finely chopped
fresh flat-leaf parsley

2 Tbsp finely chopped fresh cilantro

fine sea salt and freshly ground pepper

BEET KETCHUP

2 medium beets, trimmed
and peeled (9 oz)

½ cup apple cider vinegar

2 Tbsp minced yellow or red onion

1 Tbsp coconut sugar

¼ tsp fine sea salt

¼ tsp ground coriander

pinch of ground cloves

1. To make the beet ketchup, preheat the oven to 400°F. Cut each beet into 8 pieces, then arrange in a small baking dish with ⅓ cup water and cover. Roast until soft, about 45 minutes. Transfer the beets and their cooking liquid to a small saucepan and stir in the remaining ketchup ingredients. Bring to a boil over medium-high heat, then reduce the heat to low, partially cover the pan, and simmer, stirring occasionally, until the liquid reduces slightly and the beets are very soft, about 25 minutes. (If the liquid reduces before the beets are very soft, add a little boiling water to the pan and continue to cook.) Transfer the mixture to a blender or food processor and process to a smooth purée, adding a little water if needed to achieve your desired consistency. Taste and adjust the seasoning. Transfer to an airtight container. Let cool to room temperature, then refrigerate for up to 1 week.

2. To make the fries, position 2 oven racks evenly in the middle of the oven and preheat the oven to 425°F. Trim the ends of the sweet potato, cut it lengthwise into ½-inch-thick slabs, then stack the slabs and cut into ½-inch-wide batons. Transfer to a large, wide bowl. Cut the carrots in half crosswise, then cut each half into quarters to form roughly ½-inch-wide batons. Cut the parsnips in half lengthwise, then cut each half lengthwise into ½-inch-wide batons.

Root Veggie Fries (cont.)

3. Toss the vegetables with the oil and coat evenly. Divide the vegetables between 2 large rimmed baking sheets, with the sweet potato on one and the carrots and parsnips on the other. Arrange them in a single layer on each sheet so the pieces aren't touching.

4. Bake until the bottoms of the vegetables are golden, rotating the pans halfway through, about 13 minutes. Turn the vegetables over so they cook evenly, then continue to cook until the other side is golden brown, again rotating the pans halfway through, 6 to 9 minutes longer. Cook for 19 to 22 minutes total, until the fries are tender on the inside and deeply golden on the outside. (If you like, turn off the oven and leave the fries on the pan to stay warm for up to 10 minutes.)

5. Transfer to a serving platter, sprinkle with the chopped parsley and cilantro on top, then season with salt and pepper. Serve hot, with the beet ketchup alongside for dipping.

COMFORTED FOOD-MOOD CHEAT SHEET

Quick Tip: Choose foods that make you feel good both physically and emotionally, like a hug from the inside out.

ancient grains	maize
avocados	nuts
beans	pumpkin seeds
chickpeas	rice
cinnamon	salmon
coconut milk	strawberries
dark leafy greens	sweet potatoes
grapes	turkey
lentils	walnuts

COMFORT RITUAL

Create the Ultimate Cozy Nook

Ever heard of *hygge*?

Pronounced "hoo-gah," this Danish word means "coziness"—specifically the safe, warm, relaxed contentment that you feel inside a cozy home. Think of the scent of cookies baking in the oven. Snuggling under a thick blanket on a cold, rainy night. Or that delicious feeling of slipping into clean pajamas, fresh and warm right from the dryer.

The word hygge stems from a sixteenth-century Scandinavian word with the same root as the English word *hug*. How can you make your home feel more like a cozy, loving hug?

One idea: set up a hygge nook in your home—a super-cozy corner that's all about comfort and relaxation. Decorate it with a comfy chair and blanket, extra pillows (can you ever really have too many?), a stack of books, a favorite family photo album to bring back sweet memories, a teapot, candles, or anything else that gives you that wrapped-in-a-hug feeling.

At least once a week, take some time to nestle into your hygge nook. Dive into a book, wrap your hands around a warm mug of tea, watch the candlelight flicker, or exhale and do absolutely nothing at all. Making space for comforting moments like this is so healing for your nervous system and has a positive impact on your immune system, too.

SENSUAL

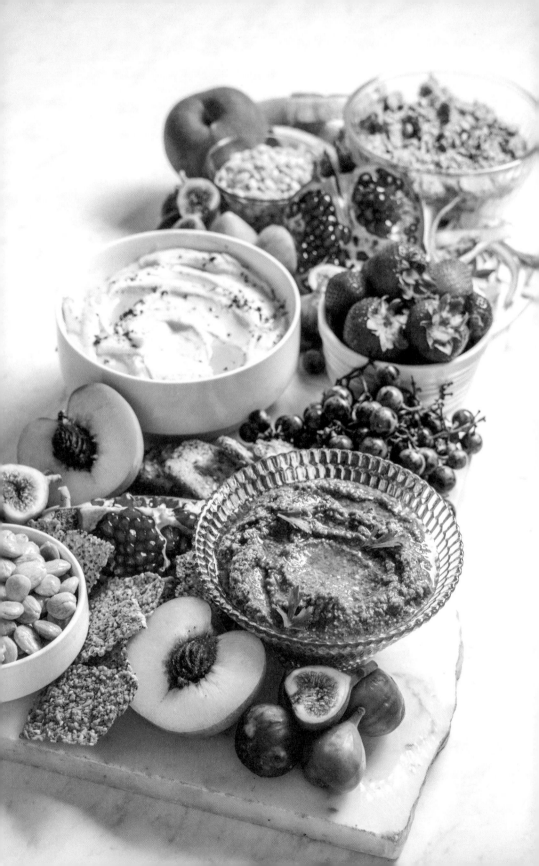

Sensual Snack Board

Want to impress your guests or a special someone? Put together an EPIC Sensual Snack Board! There are no rules; consider this as more of a guide than an actual recipe. All you need to do is a little bit of shopping and chopping to create a colorful spread. Sticking with our sensual theme, you'll toss in some of the key libido-boosting foods to get you in the mood.

VEGETABLES

Fresh veggies are key for building bulk, adding nutrients, and providing color and crunch. Vegetables such as blanched asparagus spears, sliced bell peppers, and celery sticks are great sensual choices, but check the local farmers' market to see what's in season for the best flavor. Grilled or marinated vegetables are also delicious additions to your board.

DIPS

Choose dips that highlight sensual ingredients: hummus made with garlic; avocado transformed into guacamole; basil and pine nuts in pesto. (Hint: If you're pressed for time, there are plenty of store-bought options to choose from.) Add these sexy spreads to your board in small bowls. Dust one or two with cayenne for a little extra heat.

CRACKERS AND CHIPS

Whether seeded, whole grain, grain free, or gluten free, crackers or chips add crunch and are perfect for dipping, spreading, or topping with cheese.

FRUIT

Just like vegetables, fresh seasonal fruit adds flavor, interest, and a nutritional punch to your board. Sliced strawberries, quartered fresh figs, cubes of watermelon, and bunches of red grapes are the most libido-boosting choices.

CHEESES

Depending on the size of your crowd, pick one to three dairy-based or vegan cheeses that complement the veggies, dips, crackers, and fruit on your board. Be sure to check out the innovative non-dairy, nut-based spreadable cheeses now available.

Sensual Snack Board (cont.)

SOMETHING SAVORY

A bowl of briny olives or crunchy toasted nuts is a simple way to add savory, salty flavor to your board. Almonds, pistachios, and walnuts top the sensual list.

A LITTLE SWEET

Add a touch of sweetness to the snacking experience with shards of good-quality dark chocolate, or a drizzle of honey (it's great with cheese or fruit). Or go over the top with a few small jars of Spiced Edible Chocolate Chip Cookie Dough (page 275) for an extra-sexy treat!

●●●

To assemble, gather all of your ingredients and arrange them decoratively on a wooden cutting board, a cheese board, a platter, or even a baking tray. Place the bowls with dip, spreads, nuts, and/or olives on the board first, and then array the other ingredients around them. For the most visual pop, slice fruits and vegetables into different shapes, then keep colors separate. Have fun with it, and don't worry about trying to make it perfect. Keep it simple enough that you can relax and be present with your guests or special someone!

Asparagus Salad with Pesto Vinaigrette

MAKES 4 SERVINGS

Fresh asparagus is a harbinger of spring, and roasting it turns this earthy vegetable a little sweet. As a source of folate, asparagus can help increase the histamine in our bodies, an essential component for maintaining a healthy sex drive. The pesto vinaigrette gets richness from the addition of pine nuts, another known aphrodisiac. Pine nuts contain zinc, which supports the production of sex hormones, such as testosterone and prolactin, as well as arginine, an amino acid that can help dilate blood vessels. Consider this your starting point and add whatever other vegetables you have on hand to this simple but sensual salad.

Tip: Some of my favorite springtime additions are sliced sugar snap peas, diced roasted beets, shaved baby fennel, sliced watermelon radish, and/or slices of ripe avocado.

INGREDIENTS

¼ cup plus 2 Tbsp pine nuts, lightly toasted

2 cups fresh basil leaves

3 Tbsp freshly grated Parmesan (dairy or vegan)

1 Tbsp red wine vinegar

1 Tbsp fresh lemon juice

⅓ cup plus 1 Tbsp extra-virgin olive oil, plus more if needed

Fine sea salt and freshly ground black pepper

1 lb medium-size asparagus

2 cups mixed baby lettuces or baby arugula (about 2 oz)

1. To make the pesto vinaigrette, in a food processor pulse ¼ cup pine nuts until minced. Add the basil, Parmesan, vinegar, and lemon juice. Pulse until the basil is finely chopped and all the ingredients well mixed. Scrape down the sides of the bowl. With the motor running, add 1/3 cup oil to create a smooth dressing; add a little more if needed to get the consistency you like. Transfer to a bowl. Taste and season with salt and pepper.

2. Preheat the oven to 425°F. Snap off the tough ends of the asparagus. Arrange on a rimmed parchment-lined baking sheet. Drizzle with 1 tablespoon of oil, then season lightly with salt and pepper. Roast until just barely tender, 3 to 5 minutes (depending on thickness). Transfer to a cutting board. When cool enough to handle, cut into bite-sized pieces, or leave whole if you like the look of the long spears.

3. In a bowl, toss the lettuces with about 2 tablespoons of pesto vinaigrette. Arrange the lettuces on a serving platter. Top with the asparagus. Drizzle with some of the pesto vinaigrette. Garnish with the remaining 2 tablespoons pine nuts. Serve, passing any additional pesto alongside.

Roasted Delicata Squash with Figs, Arugula, and Tahini Drizzle

MAKES 4 SERVINGS

Let's be honest: figs are the sexiest fruit out there, so it should be no surprise that they have been known as an aphrodisiac from antiquity, containing nutrients to fire up sexual stamina. Fun fact: they were even Cleopatra's favorite fruit! You can use any winter squash in this recipe—butternut, kabocha, kuri—but I like delicata because you don't have to peel it. Plus it makes a pretty presentation when roasted in rings. Add all the ingredients to a bed of arugula, a good source of zinc to improve blood flow and a popular aphrodisiac among ancient Romans and ancient Egyptians, and marry all of the flavors with an elegant lemony tahini dressing.

Tip: If using other winter squashes, be sure to peel them, scoop out the seeds, and cut into 1/2-inch-thick slices. Adjust the cooking time as needed.

SQUASH SALAD

2 lbs delicata squash

½ small red onion, halved and thinly sliced

2 Tbsp olive oil

fine sea salt and freshly ground black pepper

4 cups baby arugula

4 large, ripe fresh figs, trimmed and quartered

2 tsp toasted sesame seeds

1 Tbsp chopped fresh flat-leaf parsley

TAHINI DRESSING

¼ cup tahini

¼ cup fresh lemon juice

2 Tbsp extra-virgin olive oil

¼ tsp fine sea salt

pinch of black pepper

1. To make the tahini dressing, in a small bowl whisk together the tahini, lemon juice, olive oil, salt, and pepper. Thin with 2 tablespoons water, or enough to make a pourable consistency. Set aside.

2. Preheat the oven to 425°F. Slice the squash into 1/2 inch rounds; use a spoon to scoop out the seeds. Transfer the squash rings to one side of a large rimmed baking sheet, placing the sliced onion on the other side. Drizzle the squash and onion with the olive oil and season with salt and pepper. Toss gently to coat evenly, then spread into an even layer (again, keeping them separate).

3. Roast, stirring the onions once or twice, until the onions and squash are browned and tender, about 15 minutes for the onions and about 25 minutes

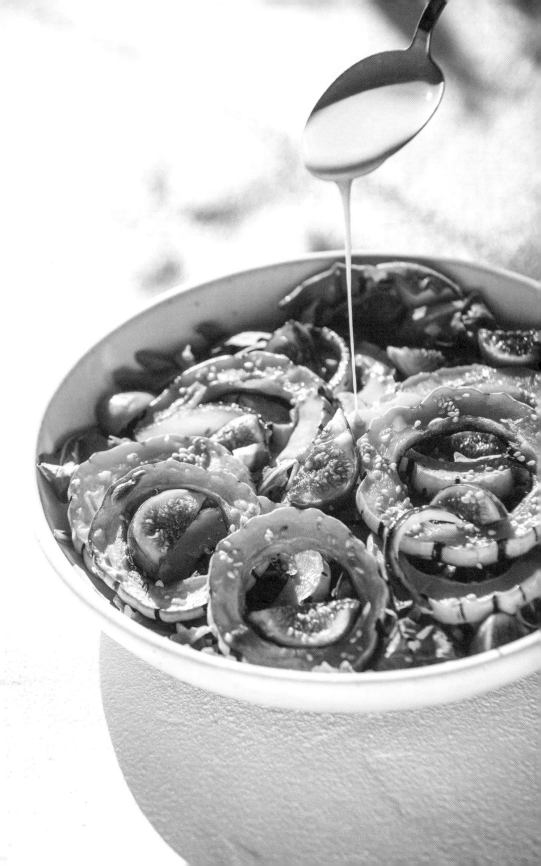

Roasted Squash with Figs (cont.)

for the squash. (When the onions are ready, transfer to a plate and continue roasting the squash.) When the squash is ready, set aside on the pan to cool slightly.

4. Spread the arugula on a serving platter. Arrange the roasted squash and onions on top in an even layer. Drizzle with some of the tahini dressing. Arrange the figs on top. Garnish with the sesame seeds and parsley and serve.

Spiced Edible Chocolate Chip Cookie Dough

MAKES 4 SERVINGS

It may shock you that a decadent dessert can be created from chickpeas, but this crave-worthy recipe is nothing short of surprising. This indulgent treat brings together several sexy ingredients: nut butter, which adds richness; maple syrup, to provide just enough sweetness; cinnamon, a warming spice used since ancient times as an aphrodisiac; ginger, which increases blood flow; and cardamom, recommended for low libido in the ancient Indian healing tradition of Ayurveda.

Tip: Keep the edible cookie dough nut-free by using sunflower butter instead of nut butter.

INGREDIENTS

1 15.5-oz can chickpeas (about 1½ cups), drained and rinsed

¼ cup almond butter or cashew butter

¼ cup maple syrup

¼ cup almond flour or oat flour

2 Tbsp almond, cashew, or oat milk

1 Tbsp ground flaxseed

1 tsp vanilla extract

½ tsp ground cinnamon

½ tsp ground ginger

¼ tsp ground cardamom

⅛ tsp baking soda

⅛ tsp fine sea salt, or to taste

½ cup chocolate chips

1. In the bowl of a food processor, combine all the ingredients except for the chocolate chips. Process until smooth, about 2 minutes, scraping down the sides with a rubber spatula as needed.

2. Transfer the mixture to a bowl. Stir in the chocolate chips. Cover and refrigerate for at least 30 minutes, then serve in small bowls or jars with a spoon. (Can be stored in an airtight container in the refrigerator for up to 5 days.)

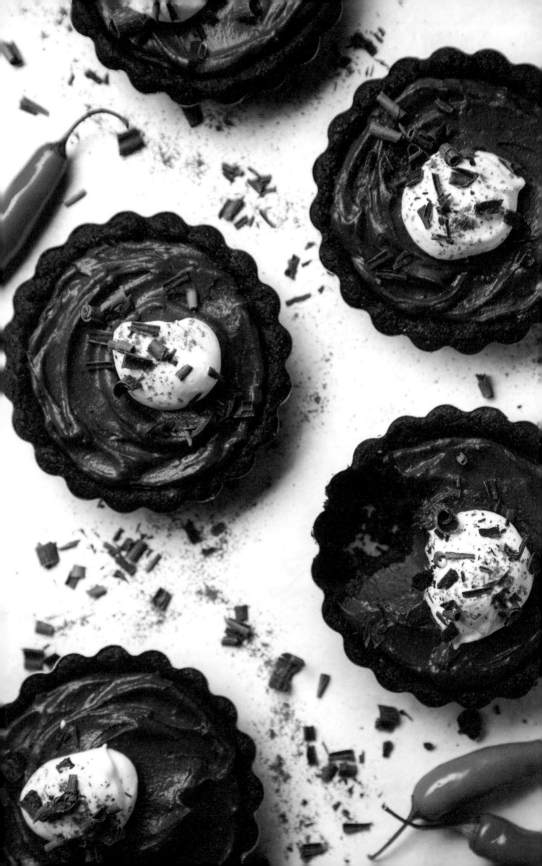

Chili-Spiced Chocolate Tartlets

MAKES ONE 9-INCH TART OR FOUR 4-INCH TARTLETS

This double chocolate tart is rich, deeply flavorful, and very sexy. Chocolate contains a compound called phenylethylamine, which triggers the release of endorphins (the same happy-making chemicals released after a great workout) and feel-good dopamine. The added chili in the custard gives it a little bit of zing. Chilies contain capsaicin, which produces heat and boosts blood flow and circulation. For a milder dessert, use one chili; add another to keep things spicy!

Tip: The crust is a great all-purpose gluten-free chocolate tart dough; to make a regular gluten-free dough, increase the tapioca flour to ½ cup and omit the cocoa powder. If you choose to use a flax egg for the filling, mix 1 tablespoon of ground flaxseed with 3 tablespoons of warm water in a small bowl. Let stand for 10 minutes until a gel-like consistency forms. You can also use chia seeds in place of flaxseed.

CRUST

½ cup white rice flour

½ cup almond flour

½ cup natural cocoa powder

3 Tbsp coconut sugar

2 Tbsp tapioca flour

½ tsp fine sea salt

⅓ cup cold coconut oil

1 large egg yolk (or 1 flax egg—see tip above)

2 Tbsp very cold water

CHILI-CUSTARD FILLING

1 13.5-oz can full-fat coconut milk

3 Tbsp natural cocoa powder, sifted

2 Tbsp cornstarch

⅓ cup coconut sugar

¼ tsp ground cinnamon

¼ tsp fine sea salt

1 or 2 dried ancho chilies, seeds removed and chilies torn into 4 pieces

3 oz dark chocolate, chopped

½ tsp vanilla extract

COCONUT WHIP

1 13.5-oz can organic coconut cream or coconut milk, chilled overnight in the refrigerator

1 Tbsp maple syrup or coconut sugar

½ tsp vanilla extract

1. To make the crust, in the bowl of a food processor, pulse the rice flour, almond flour, cocoa powder, coconut sugar, tapioca flour, and salt until evenly combined. Add the coconut oil and process until the mixture is evenly moistened, about 20 seconds. Add the egg yolk (or flax egg) and water and process until the dough is moist and easily holds together when pressed between fingertips, about 30 seconds.

Chocolate Tartlets (cont.)

2. If making 4 tartlets, grease four 4-inch tartlet pans with removable bottoms. Divide the dough into 4 equal portions. If making 1 larger tartlet, grease a 9-inch tart pan with a removable bottom. Gently ease the dough into the pan(s), pressing it into the corners and up the sides; use the base of a small glass to help you even out the dough. Place the pan(s) on a baking sheet and refrigerate for at least 30 minutes or up to overnight.

3. Preheat the oven to 375°F. Bake until the crust looks set, about 15 minutes. Transfer to a wire rack to cool.

4. To make the custard, pour the coconut milk into a saucepan and whisk to combine if it is separated. Transfer ⅓ cup of the coconut milk to a medium bowl and add the cocoa powder, cornstarch, coconut sugar, cinnamon, and salt. Whisk to a smooth paste. Set aside.

5. Add the ancho chilies to the remaining coconut milk in the saucepan. Bring to a gentle boil over medium-high heat. Remove from the heat, cover, and set aside to steep for 10 minutes.

6. Strain the coconut milk–chili mixture through a fine-mesh sieve set over the bowl with the cocoa powder paste; discard the chili. Whisk the mixture together until smooth, then transfer to the saucepan and set over medium-low heat. Bring to a simmer, stirring constantly with a whisk, until the mixture is thick, glossy, and smooth and coats the back of a spoon, about 4 minutes. Remove from the heat and add the dark chocolate and the vanilla. Stir until the chocolate is completely melted and the mixture is smooth.

7. Immediately pour the custard into the prepared tart shell(s), smoothing it into an even layer. To keep it from forming a skin, cover with parchment paper pressed directly onto the custard. Refrigerate until set and chilled completely, at least 2 hours or up to overnight.

8. To make the coconut whip, put a mixing bowl in the freezer for 15 minutes before whipping the cream. Without shaking or tipping the can of coconut milk, remove the can from the refrigerator and use a can opener to open the top. Scoop the hardened part of the coconut cream or milk into the cold mixing bowl, leaving the liquid in the bottom of the can (don't discard). Using an electric mixer, beat the chilled coconut cream, maple syrup or coconut sugar, and vanilla together until smooth, soft peaks form. If the coconut whip is chunky or overly thick, add a little of the liquid from the can to smooth it out.

9. To serve, remove the tart(let) ring(s) and base(s). Place each tartlet on an individual plate or cut the large tart into wedges and transfer to plates. Top the tart or tartlets with the coconut whip and serve.

SENSUAL FOOD-MOOD CHEAT SHEET

Quick tip: Choose foods that promote circulation and blood flow, sex hormone production, and (ahem) hydration and lubrication.

asparagus	lentils
beans	maca powder
cardamom	oysters
cinnamon	pine nuts
chilies	pumpkin seeds
dark chocolate	shrimp
figs	strawberries
garlic	watermelon
honey	whole grains

SENSUAL RITUAL

Indulge Your Senses . . . and Take a Floating Vacation

You can have a beautifully sensual, sexy life . . . even if you're not in a relationship right now. It's all about cultivating a mindset that prioritizes taking care of yourself, regardless of whom you're with.

For a fabulously sensual ritual, take a long bath. But not just any bath—make it really special. Like a floating vacation. Go completely over the top: Epsom salts to soothe sore muscles. Fragrant aromatherapy oils. Bubbles. Flower petals. Put a candle (or ten) around your bathroom. Complete the mood with soothing music. Let yourself luxuriate in the tub. Gently scrub your entire body, silently sending a simple thank-you message to each part. "Thank you, legs, for carrying me everywhere. Thank you, stomach, for being my center and holding me together . . ." The more you extend gratitude (instead of criticism) to your body, the more confident, self-assured, and sensual you will feel.

No bathtub? Create a similar experience in your shower. Research confirms that being near water, in water, or even just looking at a photo of water makes us feel better. Humans innately crave water and love being immersed in it. There's something so powerful about taking an intentional bath, shower, or swim. People have engaged in ritualistic bathing since the dawn of time, and for good reason. It shifts you!

CALM

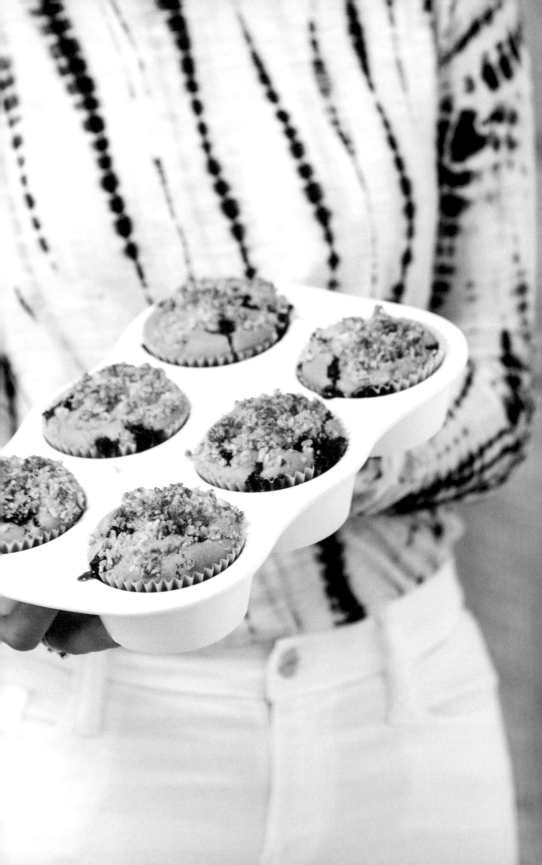

Blueberry Almond Muffins with Crunchy Nut Topping

MAKES 12 MUFFINS

Tap into the therapeutic benefits of baking with these tender, gluten-free muffins. With their high levels of antioxidants, including an abundance of vitamin C, blueberries are always a good addition for anxiety and stress relief. And the crunchy Brazil nut and almond topping adds flavor, texture, and several calming ingredients. Did you know that a single Brazil nut has a day's worth of selenium, a vitamin that has been linked to a decrease in anxiety levels and a boost in calm moods? And almonds contain magnesium, another stress-buster nutrient.

Tip: Swap out the blueberries for raspberries or chopped blackberries. Or add 1 teaspoon of finely grated lemon zest to the batter for a tangy flavor.

MUFFINS

1 cup almond flour

¾ cup brown rice flour

⅓ cup tapioca flour

2 tsp baking powder

¼ tsp baking soda

¼ tsp fine sea salt

¾ cup unsweetened almond milk or oat milk

⅓ cup maple syrup or coconut sugar

⅓ cup melted coconut oil

2 large eggs

1 tsp vanilla extract

1 cup (6 oz) fresh blueberries

CRUNCHY NUT TOPPING

⅓ cup old-fashioned rolled oats

½ cup chopped roasted Brazil nuts

⅓ cup sliced toasted almonds

3 Tbsp almond flour

2 Tbsp melted coconut oil

2 Tbsp maple syrup

¼ tsp vanilla extract

pinch of fine sea salt

A VEGAN, SUGAR-FREE VARIATION

Swap the maple syrup for 1 large, ripe, mashed banana and swap the whole eggs for two flax eggs made from 2 tablespoons ground flaxseed and 5 tablespoons warm water. (See page 277.) These make a delicious but much more crumbly and delicate muffin.

1. Preheat the oven to 375°F. Line the cups of a standard 12-cup muffin pan with paper liners.

2. To make the topping, in the bowl of a food processor, pulse the oats about 5 times, until they are slightly chopped. Add the Brazil nuts and almonds and pulse until the nuts are finely chopped but still have some texture. Add the almond flour, coconut oil, maple syrup, vanilla, and salt. Pulse until the mixture comes together. Set aside.

Blueberry Almond Muffins (cont.)

3. In a large bowl, whisk together the almond flour, rice flour, tapioca flour, baking powder, baking soda, and salt. In another bowl, whisk together the milk, maple syrup or coconut sugar, coconut oil, eggs, and vanilla. Add the wet ingredients to the dry ingredients and stir until smooth. Stir in the blueberries.

4. Using a ¼-cup measure, divide the batter between the prepared muffin cups, filling them nearly full. Top the batter with the nut topping, dividing it evenly between the muffin cups. Let the batter sit for 5 minutes in the cups, then bake until a toothpick inserted into the center comes out clean, 23 to 25 minutes. Place the pan on a rack to cool for at least 20 minutes before removing the muffins from the pan. Serve.

Popcorn with Turmeric Seasoning Blend

MAKES 2 TO 4 SERVINGS

Did you know crunchy foods can help relieve stress? So grab a fresh batch of turmeric-seasoned popcorn and eat your way to calm. Curcumin, the main active ingredient in turmeric, is reported to reduce anxiety by stimulating the release of serotonin and dopamine in the brain. To get the most benefit from turmeric, don't skip the black pepper. It increases the bioavailability of this potent herb. And be sure to wash your hands after eating and before touching anything, so the bright yellow seasoning doesn't end up on your furniture or clothes!

Tip: Add even more nutritional yeast, a deactivated yeast and good source of B vitamins, to create a cheesy flavor without any cheese.

INGREDIENTS

2 Tbsp nutritional yeast, or to taste

1 tsp ground turmeric

½ tsp garlic powder

½ tsp fine sea salt, or to taste

⅛ tsp freshly ground black pepper

2 Tbsp coconut oil or ghee

½ cup popcorn kernels

1. In a small bowl, whisk together the nutritional yeast, turmeric, garlic powder, salt, and pepper. Set aside.

2. In a large pot over medium-high heat, warm the oil or ghee. Add 3 or 4 popcorn kernels to the pot. When they pop, add the remaining kernels to the pot, spreading them in a single layer on the bottom. Cover the pot, reduce the heat to medium, and cook, shaking the pan occasionally.

3. When the popping slows to only a few pops every 10 seconds, remove the pot from the heat. Pour the popcorn into a large bowl. Sprinkle the seasonings over the popcorn and toss to coat evenly. Adjust salt to taste. Serve at once.

Colorful Chopped Fiesta Salad

Embrace the meditative quality of chopping and use the time you spend preparing the ingredients for this hearty, flavorful salad to ease into a calmer, more relaxed pace. Then let the delicious medley of protein, fiber, and healthy fats do their work, stabilizing your blood sugar and balancing your mood. Leafy greens and beans give you an ample supply of magnesium, and the colorful vegetables provide an array of phytonutrients to top it all off. The chili-lime vinaigrette adds zing and can be varied to suit your tastes. Like it spicy? Add a pinch of cayenne. Like it sweeter? Add a touch of honey. You can even swap out lemon for the lime. For extra crunch, serve the salad with crispy tortilla strips.

SALAD

4 cups baby kale, shredded kale, or mixed lettuces

1 cup cooked quinoa

1 15.5-oz can black beans, rinsed and drained (about 1½ cups cooked beans)

½ cup cooked corn kernels (fresh or frozen)

fine sea salt and freshly ground black pepper

⅓ cup chopped roasted or raw red bell peppers

4 radishes, very thinly sliced

1 cup quartered cherry tomatoes

1 ripe avocado, pitted, peeled, and thinly sliced

chopped fresh cilantro leaves, for garnish

CHILI-LIME VINAIGRETTE

½ cup avocado oil

¼ cup lime juice

1 Tbsp apple cider vinegar

1 Tbsp packed cilantro leaves

1 tsp honey (optional)

½ tsp ground chili powder, such as ancho or chipotle

¼ tsp ground cumin

¼ tsp fine sea salt

1. To make the vinaigrette, add all of the ingredients to a blender. Blend on medium-high speed until well mixed and emulsified. Transfer to a bowl.

2. Place the greens in a large bowl and drizzle with 2 tablespoons vinaigrette. Toss to coat evenly, then divide between 4 individual plates. Add the quinoa, black beans, and corn to the bowl with 2 tablespoons vinaigrette and toss to coat evenly. Season with salt and pepper. Spoon the quinoa mixture on top of the greens, dividing evenly. Top the salads with the bell peppers, radishes, cherry tomatoes, and avocado. Drizzle with a little more vinaigrette and garnish with cilantro. Serve immediately, passing any remaining vinaigrette alongside.

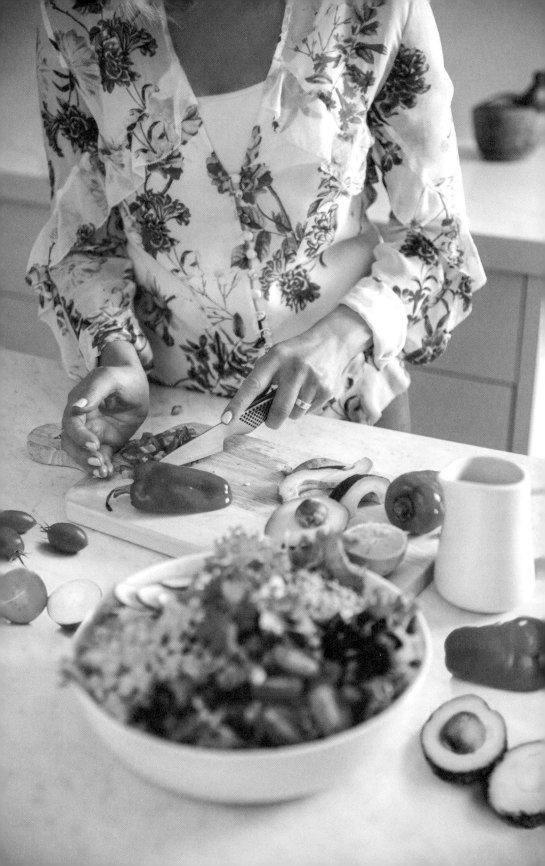

Roasted Crucifers with Tomato-Saffron Sauce and Greens

MAKES 4 TO 6 SERVINGS

This is really multiple recipes all rolled into one: a great basic tomato sauce, an easy method for roasting crucifers, such as cauliflower and broccoli, and a simple sauté of garlicky greens. Although all of these ingredients can have a calming effect, the real star of the dish is saffron. This sunshine spice has been shown to help with anxiety and depression by balancing levels of dopamine, norepinephrine, and serotonin. A little goes a long way, and it combines magically into the tomato sauce. Use fresh skinned, seeded, and chopped ripe tomatoes when they are in season in the summer. And have fun mixing up the crucifers: use all of one type or throw in some purple or yellow cauliflower, pale green Romanesco broccoli, or even broccolini!

Tip: While saffron may seem exotic, it is now more widely accessible and available. Just a few threads are all you need.

TOMATO-SAFFRON SAUCE

2 Tbsp extra-virgin olive oil

½ yellow onion, finely chopped

fine sea salt and freshly ground black pepper

½ tsp loosely packed crumbled saffron threads

1 28-oz can whole tomatoes, with juices, or equivalent amount of jarred tomatoes

¼ cup sliced green or black olives (optional)

ROASTED CRUCIFERS AND GREENS

6 cups cauliflower, broccoli, and/or Romanesco florets (about 1½ lbs)

2 Tbsp extra-virgin olive oil

fine sea salt and freshly ground black pepper

1 large clove garlic, minced

8 oz chopped fresh greens, such as collard greens, spinach, kale, or Swiss chard

2 Tbsp finely chopped fresh flat-leaf parsley, for garnish

1. To make the sauce, warm the oil in a saucepan over medium-low heat. Add the onion and a pinch of salt and cook, stirring occasionally, until tender and golden, about 4 minutes. Add the saffron and cook, stirring, until fragrant, about 30 seconds. Reduce the heat to low and add the tomatoes and their juices, crushing them into the saucepan with your hands as you add them. Add ¼ teaspoon salt and a few grinds of pepper. Increase the heat to medium-high, bring to a boil, then reduce the heat to low and simmer, partially covered, until the tomatoes are fragrant and saucy, about 30 minutes. Stir in the olives, if using, and season with more salt and pepper. Remove from the heat and cover to keep warm.

2. Preheat the oven to 425°F. Place the florets on a large rimmed baking sheet and drizzle with 1 tablespoon of oil. Season with salt and pepper. Spread into an even layer. Roast, turning the vegetables once or twice, until they are crisp-tender and nicely browned in places, about 20 minutes.

3. While the crucifers roast, make the greens. In a large, heavy skillet over medium heat, warm the remaining tablespoon of oil. Add the garlic, and when it starts to sizzle, add the greens. Season with salt and pepper and cook, stirring, until the greens are wilted and tender, 2 to 5 minutes, depending on the type of greens you are using.

4. Divide the greens between individual plates or spread on a serving platter. Top the greens with the roasted crucifers, then spoon some of the sauce over the top of the crucifers. Garnish with the parsley and serve at once. (Any leftover sauce can be stored in an airtight container in the refrigerator for up to 1 week.)

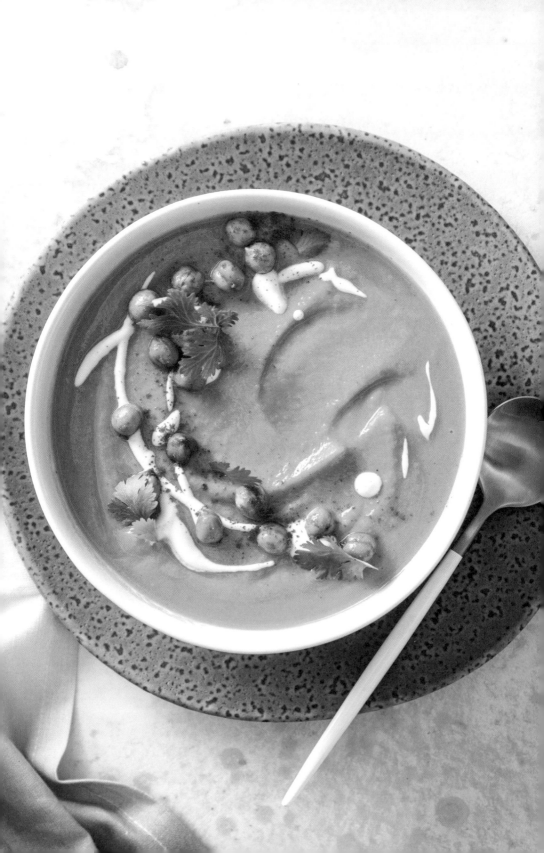

Roasted Root Vegetable and Chickpea Soup

Full of warming spices with anxiety-reducing properties, this hearty soup will flood your body with nourishment and calm. Along with root vegetables, protein-packed chickpeas create the base and do double duty as a crispy topping that is satisfying as a snack all on its own. (Trust me, I can't stop eating them!) And did you know chickpeas are also an excellent source of tryptophan? The complex carbohydrates in the soup help with the absorption of this amino acid to give you a serotonin boost. Just remember to slow down and take a few deep breaths—the ultimate stress buster!

Tip: You can use butternut squash in place of the sweet potatoes for a different variation.

INGREDIENTS

1 tsp ground cumin

1 tsp ground paprika

½ tsp ground coriander

fine sea salt and freshly ground black pepper

1 sweet potato (about ¾ lb), peeled and cut into 1-inch chunks

2 medium parsnips (about ½ lb), peeled and cut into 1-inch chunks

2 carrots (about ½ lb), peeled and cut into 1-inch chunks

3 Tbsp extra-virgin olive oil or avocado oil

1 15.5-oz can chickpeas (about 1½ cups)

½ yellow onion, finely chopped

1 clove garlic, minced

5 cups low-sodium vegetable broth or water, plus more as needed

about ¼ cup coconut cream, for serving

about ¼ cup chopped fresh cilantro, for garnish

1. Preheat the oven to 425°F. In a small bowl, stir together the cumin, paprika, coriander, 1 tsp salt, and ¼ teaspoon pepper. Pile the sweet potato, parsnips, and carrots onto a large rimmed baking sheet and drizzle with 1 tablespoon oil. Toss to coat evenly, then sprinkle with 2 teaspoons spice mixture. Toss again, then spread the vegetables into an even layer. Roast, turning a few times during cooking, until the vegetables are browned and tender, about 25 minutes.

2. Drain and rinse the chickpeas in a colander. Set aside 1 cup chickpeas in a bowl. Spread the remaining (you should have about ½ cup) on a paper towel and pat completely dry. Set aside.

3. In a saucepan or Dutch oven over medium heat, warm 1 tablespoon oil. Add the onion and garlic, then sauté, stirring occasionally, until softened and starting to turn golden, about 5 minutes. Add the reserved 1 cup

Root Vegetable and Chickpea Soup (cont.)

chickpeas and cook, stirring, to warm through, 1 or 2 minutes. Add the stock or water and increase the heat to high, bring to a boil, then reduce the heat to medium-low. Add the roasted vegetables, stir to combine, and simmer for 10 minutes.

4. Using an immersion blender, purée the soup until smooth. Alternatively, purée the soup in a blender or food processor, processing in batches if necessary. Add additional stock or water to get the consistency you like. Return to the saucepan and place over low heat to warm gently while you make the crispy chickpeas.

5. To make the crispy chickpeas, place a small rimmed baking sheet in the oven to heat for 5 minutes. Place the reserved chickpeas in a bowl and sprinkle with 1 teaspoon spice mixture. Carefully pour 1 tablespoon oil onto the baking sheet. Return to the oven for a few minutes to make sure the oil is very hot, then carefully spoon the chickpeas onto the baking sheet, spreading them into a single, even layer. Roast, stirring once or twice, until crisp and golden, about 15 minutes.

6. Ladle the soup into bowls, swirl a dollop of coconut cream on top, and garnish with the crispy chickpeas and cilantro. Serve warm.

CALM FOOD-MOOD CHEAT SHEET

Quick tip: Choose foods with soothing, grounding, and anti-inflammatory properties.

almonds	fatty fish
bananas	lavender
blueberries	lentils
Brazil nuts	mushrooms
CBD	tulsi tea (holy basil)
chamomile	saffron
chickpeas	turkey
dark chocolate	turmeric

CALM RITUAL

Take Three Deep Breaths

Some weeks are so hectic that you need instant ways to create calm. Yoga works. Meditation is great. A lavender-infused bath feels ultra-relaxing. But in the midst of an overwhelming and busy day, it may not be feasible to take more than a few minutes to find ways to destress. As simple as it sounds, connecting to your breath is game changing. You build a barrier between what's happening around you and reconnect to what's going on within you.

Instead of stressing even more about time-consuming activities to release anxiety, start a ritual of taking three deep breaths before eating. It will get you into the habit of understanding how powerful your breath can be. And the good news is that you can come back to deep breathing at any moment. Simply inhale and exhale. If you're feeling really frazzled, try to slow down your breathing. Inhale for a slow count of three, thinking inside your mind, "One . . . two . . . three." Then exhale with that same slow-motion pace. Immediate calm. Doesn't that feel so much better?

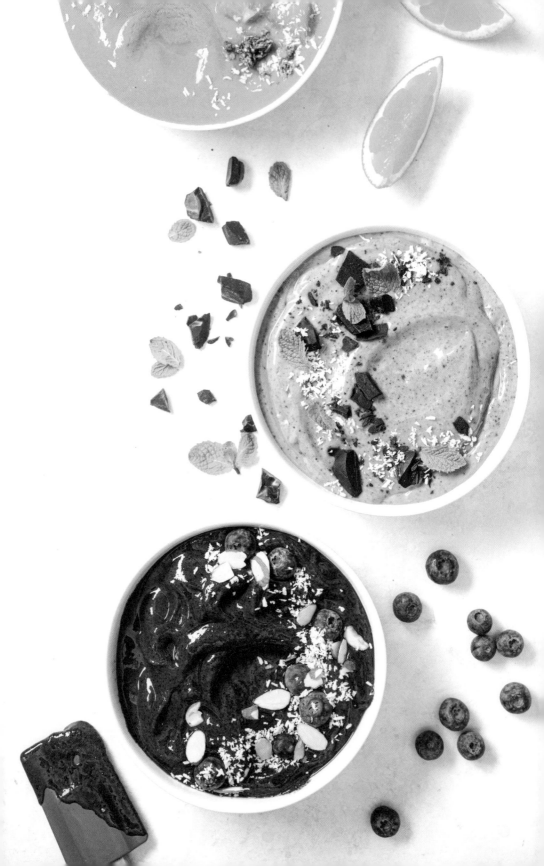

Choose Your Mood Smoothie Bowls

MAKES 1 SERVING

Smoothies and smoothie bowls are a foolproof way to pack mood-boosting ingredients and an abundance of nutrient-dense foods into your day. Even if you're strapped for time and don't consider yourself a cook, you can pull out the blender and toss in a handful of veggies, frozen fruit, healthy fat, and protein to whip up a balanced meal or snack. My younger son, Daniel, started making himself smoothies from a young age. Now, he follows this basic formula and comes up with the most drool-worthy and creative combinations. Once you get the hang of it, you won't even need to measure, and you can choose ingredients to fit your desired mood.

Tip: I prefer smoothie bowls over smoothies, as it feels more satisfying to add in texture and crunch with the toppings and eat with a spoon. For a smoothie in a glass, add more liquid to get a thinner consistency.

SMOOTHIE BOWL BASE

½ cup plant-based milk (adjust amount for desired thickness)

1 cup chopped spinach or other chopped greens of choice

1 scoop plant-based protein powder, 2 Tbsp hemp seeds, or 1 serving collagen

pinch of fine sea salt

1. Add all ingredients to a high-speed blender and blend until smooth. Next, choose a mood from the lists below and add those ingredients to the blender with the base. Blend until smooth. Serve in a bowl, add toppings of choice, grab a spoon, and dig in!

HAPPY

1 frozen banana, peeled and sliced

¼ large avocado, peeled and sliced

2 Tbsp fresh mint leaves or ⅛ tsp mint extract

1 Tbsp cacao nibs (add last and blend just to combine)

TAKE IT UP A NOTCH

1 tsp spirulina, 1 tsp matcha powder, or ½ to 1 tsp maca powder (optional; see package directions)

FOCUSED

1 cup frozen mango cubes

¼ large avocado,
peeled and sliced

1 Tbsp fresh lime juice

1 tsp finely grated lime zest

TAKE IT UP A NOTCH

1 tsp matcha powder or 2 tsp chia seeds (optional)

RADIANT

1 cup chopped frozen pineapple

¼ cup peeled chopped kiwi

¼ large avocado, peeled and sliced

2 Tbsp chopped fresh cilantro

TAKE IT UP A NOTCH

1 tsp peeled and grated fresh ginger
and/or 1 tsp camu camu powder (optional)

STRONG

1 orange, peeled, seeded,
chopped, and frozen

½ frozen banana,
peeled and sliced

½ cup frozen cauliflower rice

½ to 1 tsp grated fresh turmeric

½ tsp vanilla extract

TAKE IT UP A NOTCH

1 tsp peeled and grated fresh ginger and/or 1 tsp orange zest (optional)

COMFORTED

½ cup cooked mashed
sweet potato, frozen

½ cup frozen cauliflower rice

1 Tbsp almond butter
or cashew butter

1 Medjool date, pitted and chopped

1 tsp peeled and grated fresh ginger

½ tsp ground cinnamon

TAKE IT UP A NOTCH

2 tsp flaxseeds and/or ⅛ tsp freshly grated nutmeg (optional)

SENSUAL

1 cup frozen raspberries

½ frozen banana,
peeled and sliced

1 Tbsp almond butter or cashew butter

1 Tbsp cocoa or cacao powder

½ tsp vanilla extract

TAKE IT UP A NOTCH

½ tsp maca powder (optional; see package directions)

CALM

1 cup frozen blueberries

½ frozen banana,
peeled and sliced

½ cup chopped zucchini
(about ½ medium zucchini),
steamed and then frozen

¼ large avocado, peeled and sliced

TAKE IT UP A NOTCH

1 serving ashwagandha powder (optional)

Topping Ideas

Toppings are an excellent way to add texture, crunch, and additional mood-boosting ingredients.

- banana slices
- bee pollen
- cacao nibs
- cinnamon
- fresh berries
- fresh mint
- goji berries
- granola
- hemp seeds
- nuts
- shredded coconut

YOUR FOOD STORY LEGACY

In some way, shape, or form, we're all part of a big, interconnected web. Finding peace with food doesn't just affect you; it affects everyone around you.

Rewriting your food story positively impacts your relationships, your career, and your family. It improves your energy, your productivity, and your conversations. It enhances your confidence, your passion, and your purpose. By becoming the hero of your food story, you upgrade the quality of your life, infusing it with joy and ease that are infectious to those around you.

Healing one food story creates a ripple effect to help heal all our food stories. When we gather around our tables and celebrate food, we change the collective conversation not just for ourselves but for our children and future generations, too. It starts right now with you!

Here's to rewriting the way we eat, think, and live.

Elise

ACKNOWLEDGMENTS

Food Story is the book that I have been writing most of my life, and I couldn't have come to this place without the support, encouragement, and creativity of many people.

To my parents, Beverly and Herbert, thank you for being my biggest, most supportive fans and for teaching me the value of family dinner. I may not have appreciated it back then, but now it's a tradition that I am proud to carry on.

To my sister, Tracy, and brother, Robert, my OG food story family, thanks for all the good memories of wedging our hands in the locked fridge at night and goofing off at the kitchen table.

To my guys, Steven, Noah, and Daniel: there is a long list of reasons to thank you, but most importantly, thank you for being on this food story journey together as a family, for helping create meals that are memorable and in which everyone plays a role. In our house, there's no such thing as too many cooks in the kitchen.

To Monty and Cadence, my adorable golden retrievers, who sat under my feet (and kept me sane) as I wrote every word of this book: thank you for reminding me to get up from my desk and head outside to clear my head. You will always be my favorite writing and cuddle buddies.

To Valerie Gangas, thank you for being my spiritual partner in crime. I'm so blessed to call you my friend and even more grateful to have you on speed dial.

To Victoria Erickson, I will always appreciate you for teaching me how to feel words in my body and get into my flow state.

To Michelle ni Thuama, thank you for taking care of so many details behind the scenes and for listening to my (long) voice messages all along. I'm happy for you and your next chapter.

To my fierce agent, Coleen O'Shea, I'm honored to have you as my advocate. Thank you for guiding me through the entire publishing process. Your professionalism and dedication are unmatched.

To Linda Sivertsen, for believing in my ideas since day one and providing the most beautiful retreat experience to get clarity on this book.

To Alexandra Franzen, thank you for rescuing me when I couldn't look at my proposal any longer. You have a special gift for making everything feel simple and stress free.

To Julia Pastore, I could not have done this without you. Thank you for being the most thoughtful sounding board and for being extremely patient when I "marinated" before sending you a draft. You kept me organized with every single detail throughout the entire writing process.

To my editor at Sounds True, Diana Ventimiglia, I knew when you shared your food story with me on our first call that we were meant to be. Thank you for your continued enthusiasm every step of the way.

A special thanks to the rest of the team at Sounds True, from Jade Lascelles patiently guiding me through the production process, to Karen Polaski and Linsey Dodaro translating my ideas into an impeccable design, to Kira Roark and Nick Small of marketing and publicity spreading the *Food Story* message far and wide, and everyone else who helped me publish the book of my dreams.

To my talented photographer, Jennifer Chase, thank you for bringing my vision to life and creating the most magical visual storytelling imaginable. You have been such a blast to work with since day one.

To Nichole Bryant, my creative food stylist, thank you for creating such visual depth to the dishes. I know how much you appreciated working with these plant-based recipes.

To Giulietta Pinna of Limonata Creative, you're the coolest prop stylist and a wiz at translating ideas into art.

To Kelly Dolan, thank you for upgrading my look and helping me feel good at my photo shoot.

To Kim Laidlaw, a hug and immense gratitude for helping me take these recipes and make them truly next level. I look forward to cooking (and eating!) a meal together.

To Ruth Enckleve, my unofficial recipe tester, thank you for stepping in and navigating the grocery stores to buy all the ingredients in the middle of a global pandemic.

Finally, to my beautiful community, from my clients to my social media family to my email subscribers to my *Once Upon a Food Story* podcast listeners. I never imagined that I would reach so many incredible openhearted and open-minded people as I spread my food story message around the world. Not a day goes by that I don't pinch myself and appreciate each and every one of you. Your comments, emails, messages, and food stories inspire me daily. This book is because of you!

NOTES

PART 1: DISCOVER YOUR FOOD STORY

Chapter 2: Identify Your Food Story

1. Gert-Jan De Muynck et al., "The Effects of Feedback Valence and Style on Need Satisfaction, Self-Talk, and Perseverance among Tennis Players: An Experimental Study," *Journal of Sports and Exercise Psychology* 39, no. 1 (2017): 67–80, doi.org/10.1123/jsep.2015-0326; Yannis Theodorakis et al., "Self-Talk in a Basketball-Shooting Task," *Perceptual and Motor Skills* 92, no. 1 (2001): 309–15, doi.org/10.2466/PMS.92.1.309-315.

2. Alison Wood Brooks, "Get Excited: Reappraising Pre-Performance Anxiety as Excitement," *Journal of Experimental Psychology: General* 143, no. 3 (June 2014): 1144–58, doi.org/10.1037/a0035325.

3. Signy Sheldon and Julia Donahue, "More Than a Feeling: Emotional Cues Impact the Access and Experience of Autobiographical Memories," *Memory and Cognition* 45, no. 5 (2017): 731–44, doi.org/10.3758/s13421-017-0691-6.

4. Brenda Patoine, "The Abused Brain: Neural Adaptation, Resilience, and Compensation in Childhood Maltreatment," Dana Foundation, October 9, 2018, dana.org/article/the-abused-brain/.

PART 2: RELEASE WHAT NO LONGER SERVES YOU

Chapter 5: Release Your Old Food Story

1. Maria Konnikova, "What's Lost as Handwriting Fades," *New York Times*, June 2, 2014, nytimes.com/2014/06/03/science/whats-lost-as-handwriting-fades.html; Pam A. Mueller and Daniel M Oppenheimer, "The Pen is Mightier Than the Keyboard: Advantages of Longhand over Laptop Note Taking," *Psychological Science* 25, no. 6 (2014): 1159–68, doi.org/10.1177/0956797614524581.

Chapter 6: Quiet the Food Noise

1. "The Nielsen Total Audience Report: Q1 2018," Nielsen, July 31, 2018, nielsen.com/us/en/insights/report/2018/q1-2018-total-audience-report/.

2. Caitlin St. John, "Body Issues Begin as Early as Age 5," *Parents*, February 18, 2015, parents.com/health/parents-news-now/body-image-issues-begin -as-early-as-age-5/.

Chapter 7: Don't Bring Stress to the Table

1. Marc David, *The Slow Down Diet: Eating for Pleasure, Energy, and Weight Loss*, 10th anniversary ed. (Rochester, VT: Healing Arts Press, 2015), 19.

2. Rozalyn Simon et al., "Mantra Meditation Suppression of Default Mode Beyond an Active Task: A Pilot Study," *Journal of Cognitive Enhancement* 1, no. 2 (2017): 219–27, doi.org/10.1007/s41465-017-0028-1.

PART 3: RECONNECT WITH YOUR BODY

Chapter 8: Invite Yourself to Dinner

1. John Anderer, "'Zombie Eating': 88% of Adults Dine while Staring at a Screen, Survey Finds," Study Finds, July 24, 2019, studyfinds.org/zombie -eating-88-percent-adults-dine-while-staring-at-screen-survey-finds/.

2. Ricky Maughan, "One in Three Americans Can't Eat Without Their Phone," *New York Post*, January 23, 2018, nypost.com/2018/01/23 /one-in-three-americans-cant-eat-without-their-phone/.

3. Joshua S. Rubinstein, David E. Meyer, and Jeffrey E. Evans, "Executive Control of Cognitive Processes in Task Switching," *Journal of Experimental Psychology: Human Perception and Performance* 27, no. 4 (2001): 763–97, doi.org/10.1037//0096-1523.27.4.763.

4. Sylvain Charron and Etienne Koechlin, "Divided Representation of Concurrent Goals in the Human Frontal Lobes," *Science* 328, no. 5976 (April 2010): 360–63, doi.org/10.1126/science.1183614.

Chapter 9: Use Food to Boost Your Mood

1. Emmanuelle di Tomaso, Massimiliano Beltramo, and Daniele Piomelli, "Brain Cannabinoids in Chocolate," *Nature* 382 (1996): 677–78, doi.org/10.1038/382677a0.

2. Elizabeth R. Bertone-Johnson, Massimiliano Beltramo, and Daniele Piomelli, "Vitamin D Intake from Foods and Supplements and Depressive Symptoms in a Diverse Population of Older Women," *American Journal of Clinical Nutrition* 94, no. 4 (2011): 1104–12, doi.org/10.3945/ajcn.111.017384.

3. Claire T. McEvoy et al., "Neuroprotective Diets Are Associated with Better Cognitive Function: The Health and Retirement Study," *Journal of the American Geriatrics Society* 65, no. 8 (2017): 1857–62, doi.org/10.1111/jgs.14922; Almudena Sánchez-Villegas et al., "A Longitudinal Analysis of Diet Quality Scores and the Risk of Incident Depression in the SUN Project," *BMC Medicine* 13, no. 1 (September 2015): 197, doi.org/10.1186/s12916-015-0428-y.

4. Seanna E. McMartin, Felice N. Jacka, and Ian Colman, "The Association Between Fruit and Vegetable Consumption and Mental Health Disorders: Evidence from Five Waves of a National Survey of Canadians," *Preventive Medicine* 56, no. 3–4 (March 2013): 225–30, doi.org/10.1016/j.ypmed.2012.12.016.

5. Matthew R. Hilimire, Jordan E. DeVylder, and Catherine A. Forestell, "Fermented Foods, Neuroticism, and Social Anxiety: An Interaction Model," *Psychiatry Research* 228, no. 2 (August 2015): 203–8, doi.org/10.1016/j.psychres.2015.04.023; Alper Evrensel and Mehmet Emin Ceylan, "The Gut-Brain Axis: The Missing Link in Depression," *Clinical Psychopharmacology and Neuroscience* 13, no. 3 (December 2015): 239–44, doi.org/10.9758/cpn.2015.13.3.239.

6. Rita Haapakoski et al., "Cumulative Meta-analysis of Interleukins 6 and 1ß, Tumour Necrosis Factor α, and C-reactive Protein in Patients with Major Depressive Disorder," *Brain, Behavior, and Immunity* 49 (October 2015): 206–15, doi.org/10.1016/j.bbi.2015.06.001.

7. Lauren M. Young et al., "A Systematic Review and Meta-Analysis of B Vitamin Supplementation on Depressive Symptoms, Anxiety, and Stress: Effects on Healthy and 'At-Risk' Individuals," *Nutrients* 11, no. 9 (September 2019): 2232, doi.org/10.3390/nu11092232.

8. Anne Marie Uwitonze and Mohammed S. Razzaque, "Role of Magnesium in Vitamin D Activation and Function," *Journal of the American Osteopathic Association* 118, no. 3 (March 2018): 181–89, doi.org/10.7556/jaoa.2018.037.

9. Elizabeth E. Devore et al., "Dietary Intakes of Berries and Flavonoids in Relation to Cognitive Decline," *Annals of Neurology* 72, no. 1 (July 2012): 135–43, doi.org/10.1002/ana.23594.

10. Lawrence E. Williams and John A. Bargh, "Experiencing Physical Warmth Promotes Interpersonal Warmth," *Science* 322, no. 5901 (October 24, 2008): 606–7, doi.org/10.1126/science.1162548.

11. Christopher Dana Lynn, "Hearth and Campfire Influences on Arterial Blood Pressure: Defraying the Costs of the Social Brain Through Fireside Relaxation," *Evolutionary Psychology: An International Journal of Evolutionary Approaches to Psychology and Behavior* 12, no. 5 (November 2014): 983–1003, doi.org/10.1177/147470491401200509.

12. David Benton, "Selenium Intake, Mood, and Other Aspects of Psychological Functioning," *Nutritional Neuroscience* 5, no. 6 (November 2002): 363–74, doi.org/10.1080/1028415021000055925.

13. Case Adams, "Chamomile for Clinical Depression and Anxiety," Journal of Plant Medicines, August 13, 2014, updated October 16, 2019, plantmedicines.org/chamomile-relaxes-fights-anxiety-and-depression/.

14. Heather Ann Hausenblas et al., "Saffron (*Crocus sativus L.*) and Major Depressive Disorder: A Meta-Analysis of Randomized Clinical Trials," *Journal of Integrative Medicine* 11, no. 6 (November 2013): 377–83, doi.org/10.3736/jintegrmed2013056; M. Agha-Hosseini et al., "*Crocus sativus L.* (Saffron) in the Treatment of Premenstrual Syndrome: A Double-Blind, Randomised, and Placebo-Controlled Trial," *BJOG: An International Journal of Obstetrics and Gynaecology* 115, no. 4 (March 2008): 515–19, doi.org/10.1111/j.1471-0528.2007.01652.x.

Chapter 10: How Do You Want to Feel?

1. Fabrice Dosseville, Sylvain Laborde, and Nicolas Scelles, "Music During Lecture: Will Students Learn Better?," *Learning and Individual Differences* 22, no. 2 (April 2012): 258–62, doi.org/10.1016/j.lindif.2011.10.004; Devarajan Sridharan et al., "Neural Dynamics of

Event Segmentation in Music: Converging Evidence for Dissociable Ventral and Dorsal Networks," *Neuron* 55, no. 3 (August 2007): 521–32, doi.org/10.1016/j.neuron.2007.07.003.

PART 4: WRITE YOUR NEW FOOD STORY

Chapter 11: Make Yourself THE Priority

1. "More Sleep Would Make Most Americans Happier, Healthier, and Safer," American Psychological Association, February 2014, apa.org/research /action/sleep-deprivation.aspx.

2. "1 in 3 Adults Don't Get Enough Sleep," Centers for Disease Control and Prevention, February 18, 2016, cdc.gov/media/releases/2016/p0215 -enough-sleep.html.

3. Angela Smith Lillehei et al., "Effect of Inhaled Lavender and Sleep Hygiene on Self-Reported Sleep Issues: A Randomized Controlled Trial," *Journal of Alternative and Complementary Medicine* 21, no. 7 (July 2015): 430–38, doi.org/10.1089/acm.2014.0327.

4. Danielle F. Shanahan et al., "Nature-Based Interventions for Improving Health and Wellbeing: The Purpose, the People, and the Outcomes," *Sports* 7, no. 6 (June 2019): 141, doi.org/10.3390/sports7060141; Gregory N. Bratman et al., "Nature Reduces Rumination and sgPFC Activation," *Proceedings of the National Academy of Sciences* 112, no. 28 (July 2015): 8567–72, doi.org/10.1073/pnas.1510459112.

5. MaryCarol R. Hunter, Brenda W. Gillespie, and Sophie Yu-Pu Chen, "Urban Nature Experiences Reduce Stress in the Context of Daily Life Based on Salivary Biomarkers," *Frontiers in Psychology* 10 (2019): 722, doi.org/10.3389/fpsyg.2019.00722.

6. Min-Sun Lee et al., "Interaction with Indoor Plants May Reduce Psychological and Physiological Stress by Suppressing Autonomic Nervous System Activity in Young Adults: A Randomized Crossover Study," *Journal of Physiological Anthropology* 34, no. 1 (April 2015): 21, doi.org/10.1186/s40101-015-0060-8.

7. Jory MacKay, "Screen Time Stats 2019: Here's How Much You Use Your Phone During the Workday," RescueTime Blog, March 21, 2019, blog.rescuetime.com/screen-time-stats-2018/.

8. Gwen Dwar, "The Cognitive Benefits of Play," Parenting Science, last modified February 2014, parentingscience.com/benefits-of-play.html.

9. Jennifer Wallace, "Why It's Good for Grown-Ups to Go Play," *Washington Post*, May 20, 2017, washingtonpost.com /national/health-science/why-its-good-for-grown-ups-to-go-play /2017/05/19/99810292-fd1f-11e6-8ebe-6e0dbe4f2bca_story.html.

10. Jennifer E. Stellar et al., "Positive Affect and Markers of Inflammation: Discrete Positive Emotions Predict Lower Levels of Inflammatory Cytokines," *Emotion* 15, no. 2 (April 2015): 129–33, doi.org/10.1037/emo0000033.

11. "The Benefits of Meatless Monday: For the Planet," Meatless Monday: The Monday Campaigns, mondaycampaigns.org/meatless-monday/benefits.

12. Ibid.

13. Ibid.

14. Joy C. Rickman et al., "Nutritional Comparison of Fresh, Frozen, and Canned Fruits and Vegetables II: Vitamin A and Carotenoids, Vitamin E, Minerals, and Fiber," *Journal of the Science of Food and Agriculture* 87, no. 7 (May 2007): 1185–96, doi.org/10.1002/jsfa.2824.

Chapter 12: Pick Up the Pen

1. Sarah Milne et al., "Combining Motivational and Volitional Interventions to Promote Exercise Participation: Protection Motivation Theory and Implementation Intentions," *British Journal of Health Psychology* 7, no. 2 (May 2002): 163–84, doi.org/10.1348/135910702169420.

RECIPE INDEX

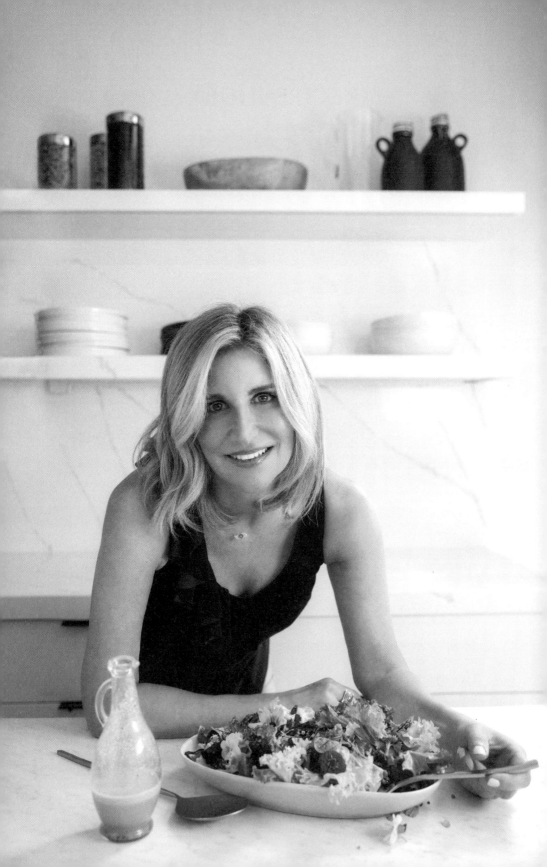

ABOUT THE AUTHOR

Elise Museles is a certified eating psychology and nutrition expert, creator of the Food Story Method and platform, and host of the popular podcast *Once Upon a Food Story*. As an author, speaker, and mind-body eating coach, Elise's mission is to empower people to create a healthier relationship with food and their bodies by changing what's on their plate—and what's in their minds.

After working as an attorney with the US Department of Justice, Elise made a career pivot to pursue her passion and became certified as a Holistic Health Coach from the Institute for Integrative Nutrition, an eating psychology coach from the Institute for the Psychology of Eating, an integrative nutrition expert from Purchase College, State University of New York, and a plant-based nutrition expert from eCornell. She's also a grant recipient for a program she developed and taught, *Cook INN Together*, at the National Institutes of Health.

Elise serves on the board of directors of Environmental Working Group, the nation's leading organization for making safer choices and creating positive momentum for American health/wellness initiatives. Her advice and recipes have been featured in many renowned wellness publications and media sources, including the bestselling books *Gutbliss* and *The Microbiome Solution, The Reducetarian Solution, The Courage to Rise, O, The Oprah Magazine, Health, Self, Forbes, ELLE*, the *Washington Post*, Well+Good, *Elite Daily*, The Chalkboard, *Women's Health*, and mindbodygreen, among others. She's appeared on *Good*

Morning Washington, WTOP Radio, the *Dr. Taz Show* on RadioMD, and other television and radio programs. Elise is the bestselling author of *Whole Food Energy: 200 All Natural Recipes to Help You Prepare, Refuel, and Recover.*

In her down time, Elise can be found playing in nature with her two golden retrievers, practicing Vinyasa yoga, or cooking colorful, mood-boosting meals for her husband and two sons—all amazing cooks as well! Connect with Elise on Instagram, listen to her podcast *Once Upon a Food Story*, and visit her website elisemuseles.com for advice and inspiration (plus mouthwatering photos) to change the way you eat, think, and live.

ABOUT SOUNDS TRUE

Sounds True is a multimedia publisher whose mission is to inspire and support personal transformation and spiritual awakening. Founded in 1985 and located in Boulder, Colorado, we work with many of the leading spiritual teachers, thinkers, healers, and visionary artists of our time. We strive with every title to preserve the essential "living wisdom" of the author or artist. It is our goal to create products that not only provide information to a reader or listener but also embody the quality of a wisdom transmission.

For those seeking genuine transformation, Sounds True is your trusted partner. At SoundsTrue.com you will find a wealth of free resources to support your journey, including exclusive weekly audio interviews, free downloads, interactive learning tools, and other special savings on all our titles.

To learn more, please visit SoundsTrue.com/freegifts or call us toll-free at 800.333.9185.

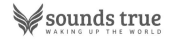